Stress and Your Heart

STRESS

and Your Heart

by Fred Kerner

With an introduction by Hans Selye, M. D.

AN AUTHORS GUILD BACKINPRINT.COM EDITION

Stress and Your Heart

All Rights Reserved © 1961, 2000 by Fred Kerner

AN AUTHORS GUILD BACKINPRINT.COM EDITION

Published by iUniverse.com, Inc.

For information address:
iUniverse.com, Inc.
620 North 48th Street, Suite 201
Lincoln, NE 68504-3467
www.iuniverse.com

Originally published by Hawthorn Books, Inc., Publishers

ISBN: 0-595-00335-4

Printed in the United States of America

For Sam, who didn't learn in time

Acknowledgments

You and I both owe a great debt to the hundreds of medical researchers who have contributed to making heart disease a vanishing ailment. Special note must be made of the great work done by Dr. Hans Selye, work that he is continuing but, more important, work that has served as a catalyst to the research of many other medical men and will undoubtedly continue to do so for generations to come. And in offering my own thanks to Dr. Selye, I also want to pay tribute to Martha Dussault and other members of Dr. Selye's staff who went out of their way to provide material useful in the preparation of this volume. I also want to thank Paul R. Reynolds, Dr. Selye's agent, for his cooperation; Vera von Fragstein, my mother, for additional research; Mickey Swedosh, my typist, for so capably deciphering my garbled notes; and above all, my wife Sally, for suggestions and encouragement.

—F.K.

Contents

7

Introduction

There is an ever-increasing demand on the part of the public for books that explain the results of current medical research and, at the same time, translate its lessons into terms of practical applicability in everyday life. In *Stress and Your Heart*, Fred Kerner has succeeded in accomplishing both these objectives.

It is not easy to write a book of this kind. I know from experience, for I also have tried. Unfortunately, those of us who are engaged in research work and spend all our time in laboratories always think about the newest and least-well-understood details of investigation. Consequently, we become too preoccupied with minutiae to make any simple general statement about a fact without qualifying it by so many "buts" and "ifs" that the result tends to confuse, rather than clarify, the problem for the general reader. The professional writer who is not a scientist himself usually writes more comprehensibly, but often at the expense of too much compromise with scientific accuracy. Mr. Kerner's success in telling the story of the relationship between stress and heart disease is due to the fact that he avoids the most common error of popular medical books: he does not try to speak, simultaneously, the language of the doctor and of his potential patient. This volume makes no attempt to explain current stress research to physicians or scientists, but I believe it succeeds very well in outlining the essentials for the educated layman. In addition, the author makes a number of very sound recommendations concerning the way we should conduct ourselves in everyday life in order to enjoy an active and productive existence without suffering the consequences of exposure to undue stress.

There are two schools of thought about medical books for the general public. There are those who claim that we only breed hypochondriacs by talking too much about health and disease. They feel that the public cannot really understand medical problems anyway and that people become too disease-conscious by reading about medical subjects. On the other hand, public health authorities are increasingly more insistent in their efforts to familiarize the public with the early signs and causes of major maladies, because this kind of knowledge helps a person to avoid situations that may be dangerous and assists him in recognizing trouble before it is too late to seek a doctor's advice. I think that this type of information is particularly useful as regards heart disease, because here our way of life (exercise, eating habits, behavior toward other people) is so largely responsible for our predisposition to resist or succumb. Each of us can learn to do much more to protect his heart against becoming sick than the physician can after the trouble has gone too far.

In medical research, we are constantly trying to develop "models of disease" in experimental animals. These imitations of the naturally occurring maladies serve as dummies on which we can try out the possible preventive or curative effects of new procedures that may be dangerous. Until quite recently, we have had no such experimental model of stress-induced cardiac disease. A few years ago—as Mr. Kerner explains—it became possible to so prepare or sensitize experimental animals with hormones and certain salts that, in them, any kind of unaccustomed sudden stress (such as nervous excitement, cold, physical injury) elicits fatal cardiac accidents with great regularity. Using this model of stress-induced heart disease, it then became possible to study the mechanism of its production, and eventually we found various ways of preventing this type of malady in the experimental animal. Of course, a model is always only an imitation and never quite the same as the original. Hence, it would be dangerous to assume that every preventive measure that works in the model must necessarily work equally well in the natural disease. Yet a great deal of evidence has accumulated in support of the view that much of what we have learned about the factors that produce or prevent experimental heart disease in animals also applies to the corresponding maladies of man. Much of this recently acquired knowledge is of no direct value to the average reader, because it concerns methods of treatment that can be used only by the experienced physician. On the other hand, part of the newly learned lesson—perhaps the most important part—can be better applied by the patient than by his doctor, because it concerns everyday living. We have learned, for example, that the heart can do well only what it is accustomed to doing and that it must, therefore, be kept in constant training. We have shown that, in suitably sensitized rats, exposure to unaccustomed exercise can produce cardiac death; yet, under otherwise similar circumstances, this same exercise causes no ill effects if the animals are first adapted to it. Indeed, it could be demonstrated that physical training by exercise protects the heart of experimental animals even against unaccustomed injuries of other kinds—for example, against the production of heart damage by drugs that normally cause death of cardiac muscle tissue. In technical language we call this "non-specific resistance."

In this book, Mr. Kerner attempts to show how a person can profit by this knowledge. He makes specific recommendations concerning the manner in which people with different occupations, predispositions and habits can adjust their conduct so as to give the heart a chance to remain constantly fit.

I am certain that many readers will be grateful to Mr. Kerner for the advice given in this instructive and very readable book.

Hans Selye

I

Enemy of the Heart

1

A Heart in Your Future

A cure for heart disease is only a matter of time. This simple pronouncement, made a few short months ago, brought hope to countless millions of sufferers from this great killer of mankind. And it brought new hope, too, for many more millions—in this generation and in the generations to come—who seemed destined at some time or other to be stricken with heart disease.

But even if a cure should not be found, scientists are pulling ahead at such a tremendous rate with new research that they are rapidly reducing the mortality rate from this disorder. Already medical men feel that eight out of ten persons who suffer from heart attacks can survive. And these survivors are far from through with active life—the majority of them return to work. In fact, statistics show that those who remain active live the longest.

What will happen when heart disease is brought under control? Many cardiologists feel that the life span will be extended vastly. Dr. Hans Selye, whose theories of stress as they affect the heart and circulatory system are responsible for this book, himself feels that there is no known theoretical limit to human life expectancy. He points out that body tissue from animals has been kept alive and healthy for a period equivalent to one thousand years in the human scale.

"If the causes of aging can be found," says Dr. Selye, "there is no good medical reason to believe that it will not be possible for science to find some practical way of slowing the process down or even bringing it to a standstill. Aging can be regarded as a disease like any other disease; it is probably preventable or curable."

And while Dr. Selye says that he does "not mean to suggest immortality for mankind," there is no theoretical limit for the span of life. Man has often been in doubt as to *how* life should be lived, but he has never doubted that it should be—and for as long as possible. In the years since 1900 on this continent, medical developments have stretched life expectancy from 48 years to the recently announced figure of 69.8 years. This unprecedented gain of more than twenty years in little more than half a century makes bright the prospect of living out the legendary—though heretofore uncommon—three score and ten. And whereas today it may be possible to extend man's life expectancy to seventy years, there is every likelihood that it could be extended to the age of one hundred, with the added likelihood of remaining active until the age of ninety.

Can you protect yourself
against heart disease?

Does this sound incredible? It shouldn't. The truth is that medicine has made a good deal more progress toward defeating death by disease than safety authorities have made toward curbing the far smaller, but growing, number of deaths on the highway. It seems most likely that future generations can be protected from heart disease. But how can *you* protect yourself? The thesis of this book is that if you—or your doctor— can spot the beginnings of stress-decay, then your chances of preventing serious heart disease are greatly increased.

Studies have found that emotional stress is almost five times as prevalent in heart attack victims as it is in persons with normal hearts. And there are recognizable symptoms, symptoms that should warn you to check in with your family doctor. It has been definitely established by heart experts that a relationship exists between emotional stress and heart seizures. The type of person who is easygoing, not overly ambitious, and has no demanding self-image to assuage is not much troubled with emotional stress. When he does find himself in an anger-producing situation, he tends to blow off steam and get it out of his system. His opposite number, however—the potential stress victim—has a completely different type of personality. As a rule he is highly ambitious, rigidly self-disciplined, works beyond his normal capacity, and has trained himself to hold in anger and other aggressive emotions that might arouse hostility in others.

Of course, stress is very difficult to evaluate. What is stress to one person is not stress to another. For this reason, we cannot assume that our generation is under more stress than any other generation. Every generation has had tremendous stresses. There were stresses in the Napoleonic wars. It must have been very stressful trying to build a pyramid in the days of ancient Egypt. A Mayan Indian might have had his head cut off or been made a human sacrifice just because he happened to be on the wrong side of an argument, and this must have been a situation that was hyper-stressful. Yet there are demands in our civilization that were not made upon our forefathers. With the rapid speed of communication, we are being subjected to crises in a manner and with a speed that our ancestors of even a generation ago did not know.

The search
to combat stress

Unfortunately, while everyone is being made more aware of the relation between emotions and heart disease, Mark Twain's remark about the weather might well be paraphrased: Everybody talks about stress and strain and heart disease, but nobody does anything about it. Nobody, that is, but the handful of scientists who are trying to help mankind alleviate—and possibly eliminate—the situation. Their research stretches far and wide. In Dr. Selye's laboratory, artificial conditions are set up to study the effects of stress. Other researchers, working in the open air, have discovered that salmon die shortly after spawning because their glandular activity is identical with the glandular activity in man after he has been subject to excessive stress.

But while medical science is racking its collective brain, its human benefactors are lacking the common sense to benefit. Even if you do not recognize the danger signals before the heart attack, they should be recognized after the first attack. Studies show that a "mild" heart attack may be only the first milestone in a continuing process—a signal of trouble ahead. But even after such an attack, and despite the warnings of medicine, too many people are heedless of the trouble into which undue emotional stress can lead them. There are no simple solutions to the problems of life which cause undue stress and tension. What you read here can be mightily useful. Experience, too, will be a teacher. Other people can be helpful. By making the effort, you can often find new and better ways to deal with the tension of your life. But *you* must make the effort.

Like any specific disease, excess stress must be caught early. It is important to recognize the symptoms of it in your own life. You must try not to bring on emotional or physical strain by overworking any one part of your body or mind in disproportion by repeating the same action to exhaustion. And this warning should apply to your personal life equally as much as it applies to your business life. Nature likes variety. You should not allow yourself senseless repetition of the same activity when you are already exhausted. For example, it would be ridiculous if you were a machinist and then spent your leisure hours at home in a workshop bending over your workbench.

Civilization has done enough to force people into highly specialized lives, lives which may become monotonously repetitive. If you get yourself deep in a rut, you may never be able to stop and will thus suffer the results of excessive stress.

Dr. Selye, himself a vigorous, active example of how to combat stress, explains how he does this:

"At any time during the day, in discussion, at work or at play, when I begin to feel keyed up, I ask myself, 'Is this really the best thing I could do now, and is it worth the trouble of putting up resistance against counter-arguments or fatigue?' If the answer is 'No,' I just stop; or whenever this cannot be done gracefully, I simply 'float' and let things go on as they will, with a minimum of active participation."

Stress: agent
of good and evil

However, you should not always think of stress as being harmful. Perhaps one of the things that is wrong with our present civilization is that people are often protected from stress, or they strive to protect themselves from stressful situations all their lives. Therefore, they never realize the benefits of stress. Stress can be one of the productive elements of your life. The fact that your body organs react to stress, the fact that they rise to the occasion as it were, permits you to make contributions to daily living or to your work which might otherwise be impossible. Needless to say, however, excessive stress under adverse conditions can be fatal. But since some stressful situations cannot be avoided, the art is to adjust to them and, if possible, to turn them to your advantage.

The difference between stress, physical exertion, and physical overexertion should be explained. Let us take the example of you sitting at your desk. While at your desk you can experience stress but, because you are sitting, you will not experience any physical exertion. If you go out and exercise physically, however, your mind will relax and stress will be alleviated, though you now will be experiencing physical exertion. On the other hand, too much physical exertion or physical overexertion will cause stress, but stress of a different type.

Ultimately, stress is reflected in your circulatory system and eventually in your heart. Just how this happens is explained in the chapters that follow. Just what you can do to alleviate this situation as much as possible is also explained.

What affects your heart? Most doctors believe that steady physical labor or exercise strengthens a healthy heart. If the muscles of your body are fit, the muscle of your heart will be stronger. If your muscles are slack, however, your heart is less able to stand a heavy load. Heat and humidity have an effect upon the heart. As the air temperature and humidity rise, your heart works harder to keep your body temperature normal. When temperatures outside fall, your heart expends more effort to keep you warm. The colder it gets, the more work your heart must do—pumping warm blood throughout your system. At high altitudes, where the oxygen content of the air is lower, your heart has to work that much harder to extract enough oxygen to keep your tissues properly supplied.

Alcohol's effects
good and bad

In large quantities, alcohol can damage the heart muscle. If taken in limited quantities, though, it acts as a mild heart stimulant which only very slightly increases the work done by the heart. The strongest effect alcohol has on your heart is probably through your emotions. If alcohol makes you tense and angry, you should not drink. If it makes you feel relaxed and affable, many doctors feel that having a drink or two may be beneficial.

And the amount you eat affects your heart by making it work harder for a longer period after a heavy meal. Every pound of body weight that you put on your frame, over and above that which is normal for your height and build, is a strain on your heart.

27

Most hearts can do what they have been accustomed to doing. They are also equipped to cope with a fantastic number of strains, as well as to deal with great intensity of strain. But if you want your heart to last you a lifetime, you must treat it with respect.

Although there are many shelves of books filled with information about the heart and the circulatory system, there is no organ or system in the body about which man has still so much to learn. The human heart beats nearly forty million times a year. It is a pump strong enough to pump about ten tons of blood through your body in a day. If you are an engineer, or understand engineering, you could say that the heart has a rating of 1/240th of a horsepower. But not only can this pump, and the conduits through which the blood flows, get out of order—so can the blood itself. The experiments, however, that Dr. Selye and his assistants have been performing in an effort to ward off impending heart attacks are encouraging. Dr. Selye has been one hundred per cent successful in preventing heart attacks in his experimental animals. Other researchers, using the same chemical treatments as he has on animals, have reported hopeful results in the preventive treatment on humans.

We are no longer ignorant in this area of health. We realize how anger, hatred, grief, worry, fear, overexertion—all are influences most destructive of vitality. But good health is not a gift bestowed at random on this one and that one. It must be earned. The person who looks upon good health as his most important possession takes the trouble to learn how the errors and chances of un-healthiness can be avoided or reduced.

The heart's owner has his life in his own hands.

Your doctor can tell you what to do. He can provide sound medical aid. But, it is up to you whether you continue on a balanced pattern of living or whether you choose to limit your years by pressing your heart beyond its possibilities.

Medical science is doing more than its share—the rest is up to you!

II

You and Your Heart

2

The Heart:

What It Is and What It Does

The human body is a wonderful machine—and the heart is its most integral part. Where the ingenuity of man has failed, nature has succeeded: The heart is a "perpetual motion" machine. It is a bundle of muscles and is often thought to be about the size of your own fist. This is, however, not quite accurate. Medical researchers have found that the normal heart is really somewhat larger than your own fist. And it certainly doesn't look anything like your fist—actually, it looks very much like a pear with the larger end at the bottom and a little bit to the left. Another common belief is that the heart is on the left side of the body—and this is not quite accurate. The heart is behind the breastbone and only slightly to the left.

But regardless of its size, its shape, or its position, the heart is a very efficient mechanism that continues its pumping job, day and night, year after year. In fact, the heart is far more efficient than any engine that man has ever created. Scientists have discovered that the heart actually converts almost half of the fuel it has available—that is, the food you eat—into mechanical work. By comparison, a steam turbine, or even an automobile in good running order, can only convert about one quarter of the fuel that is injected into it. Therefore the mechanical efficiency of the heart is at least twice as great as that of man-made engines. Another indication of the heart's efficiency is its ability to utilize oxygen.

Why the heart
needs oxygen

As you well know, oxygen is a vital necessity to human life. Of all the oxygen you breathe, the heart gets only one-tenth. But it uses this oxygen with far more efficiency than any other organ of the body. Eighty per cent of all the oxygen the heart gets is utilized—a share of efficiency that is three times as great as any other part of the body.

34

You may logically ask why the heart needs oxygen and what it does with this oxygen. Actually, the heart needs oxygen so that its muscle fibers can help the muscles of the organ contract. As you already have discovered, the heart is really only a bundle of muscles. These muscles are in several layers and are arranged in circles and spirals. When the muscles contract, these configurations tighten. The result is that the blood is actually squeezed out of the heart into the circulatory system. If you were able to look inside your heart you would find that there are, in fact, four chambers. Two are at the top, and they are known as auricles or atria (the plural of atrium). The two at the bottom are called ventricles. The top and bottom chambers are separated by a kind of muscular valve, and the right half and left half of the heart are separated by a muscular wall. This wall prevents mixing of the blood which is being pumped into the lungs in order to get fresh oxygen with the newly refreshed blood that has come from the lungs in order to be pumped to the rest of the body.

It is obvious, then, that the heart is really a kind of double pump. What happens is that blood from the body flows into the upper right chamber and then down to the lower right chamber. When the muscle contracts, the blood from the right side of the heart is forced into the lungs, where carbon dioxide is removed and fresh oxygen is fed into the blood. Then the blood flows to the upper left-hand chamber, then down into the lower left-hand chamber, and from there it is pumped out to all parts of the body through the arterial system. The valves between the upper and lower chambers prevent the blood from being forced backward when the heart contracts to force the blood out of the pump.

While the heart has a single function—that is, to pump blood—it has to pump two different kinds of blood. The first blood is a bright red color. This is the blood that is freshly saturated with oxygen. The other blood is of a darker red hue and this is the blood that comes back from the body filled with impurities. A common misbelief is that arteries always carry the bright red blood and that veins always carry the "used" blood. This is not quite true, since arteries always carry blood *away* from the heart and veins return blood *to* the heart. Therefore, blood that is carried from the heart to the lungs—that is, the "used" blood that needs refreshing—is carried in an artery. Similarly, the re-freshed, bright red blood that flows from the lungs to the heart is carried in veins.

Telltale sounds
of your heartbeat

What about your heartbeat? Perhaps you have listened through a stethoscope to the sounds of your life-

36

pump beating. If so, what you heard probably sounds like *lubb-dub*. The second sound—the "dub"—is a shorter sound and is a little higher pitched than the first. The first sound is caused by the valves closing between the upper chambers and the lower chambers so that the blood cannot flow backward, and the noise is increased by the contraction, at almost the identical instant, of the lower chambers as they force the blood out. The second sound is made by the closing of valves in the arteries that are carrying the blood away from the heart—to the lungs, on the one hand; to the rest of the body, on the other—so that, again, the blood cannot flow backward into the heart.

The beating is not a regular one-two-one-two. There is a pause between each "lubb-dub." And this pause, which is only a fraction of a second in duration, is when the heart rests. It occurs between the time that the lower chambers of the heart have become partly filled with blood and the beginning of the next wave of blood being forced in from the upper chambers.

And so the heart continues to beat away—somewhere between seventy and eighty beats every minute and even more often during violent exercise or at moments of intense emotion. And it never rests—except for the fraction of a second between beats. Oddly enough, this fraction of a second for which the heart rests is longer than the fraction of a second during which the active work takes place in the heart. However, it is not long enough to permit the kind of relaxation that other muscles of your body need and get. Since the heart beats more than sixty times in every minute, it is obvious that the entire cycle of the heart's action takes place in less than one second. Each time the heart contracts it pushes about three ounces of blood on its way to keeping the body alive—enough blood to fill a small wine glass. This three ounces is only about 1.5 per cent of all the blood in the body. Yet mathematically it becomes obvious that every drop of blood in the body manages to pass through the heart at least once a minute. And this fact is all the more amazing when you realize that if all the blood vessels in your body were stretched out end to end they would run for 70,000 miles—enough to reach around the world about three times.

Carrying the blood
to do its work

What about these vessels that carry your blood? Are they just simply conductors of the vital fluid? Here again is a common misconception—for they are not. The blood vessels display a great ability to adapt themselves to varying conditions, and they also have a certain amount of activity on their own. There are three

38

main kinds of blood vessels—arteries, veins and capillaries. By far the largest percentage of the blood vessels in the body are capillaries. In fact, so large is the capillary system that it could hold the body's entire blood supply, which is about five quarts (or an Imperial gallon). However, only a portion of the capillary system has blood flowing through it at any particular time. The system is such that it opens and closes first in one area of the body and then in another area of the body. In this way, body tissue that requires more blood—such as in the arm or leg muscles—has a larger share of the capillary system than tissue in other parts of the body which are not as active.

The arteries are in reality the main highways of the body. They are elastic tubes of muscle fiber which are delicately lined on the inside and toughly coated on the outside. These tubes expand and contract so that they can take in more or less blood depending upon the body's demands and upon pressure that is exerted upon the body. The contraction of the arteries, and the relaxation as well, helps the pumping action of the heart so that the blood can be pushed along throughout the body and maintain its pressure. This pumping action is in harmony with the rhythm of the heart so that by checking your pulse, the heartbeat can be counted without the use of a stethoscope.

The main artery of the heart is known as the aorta. From this main highway lead off a number of other arteries—large ones that go to the head, the arms, the legs, and to various of the vital organs. The "secondary roads" that carry the blood from the arteries to the capillaries are known as arterioles. They are barely visible without a microscope. They connect up with the capillary system that is so vast that if all of the vessels of this system were opened at one time it could swallow up the entire blood supply of the body, as was pointed out earlier. Yet the individual capillaries are so tiny that the red blood cells which carry oxygen to the body have to pass through them in a sort of single file. The red blood cells are quite tiny—so tiny, in fact, that three thousand blood cells placed one atop the other would not measure an inch in height. But the walls of this capillary system are quite solid—solid enough to keep the blood from leaking out into the tissue. On the other hand, the white blood cells—the fighters against disease—as well as chemicals carried by the blood and even small amounts of liquid, can leave the blood stream by squeezing through tiny openings between the cells that make up the walls of the capillary system. The blood flows very slowly at this point. It actually takes a full minute for blood to travel through one inch of capillary tube—and this compares with blood traveling through the arterial system at a speed that has been estimated at more than forty miles an hour.

During this very slow trip through the capillary system, the oxygen and the food that the body cells require are given up by the tiny blood vessels and are fed to the tissues. Also trickling through the capillary walls is lymph, a liquid that bathes the tissue cells. And the capillaries also permit other ingredients to trickle through that are required to repair the tissues and to keep them in good running order. At the same time, waste products —carbon dioxide among others—are picked up by the blood stream as it passes through the capillary system and are carried away to be discharged when the blood again reaches the lungs.

Making blood
flow uphill

This wonderful system of blood flow has yet another amazing trick. Perhaps you have wondered how blood moving back to the lungs and heart can travel upward in the body? It is logical to assume that the blood from the upper part of the body can flow downhill from the capillaries through to the veins and then on to the heart to be refreshed with oxygen in the lungs. But what about blood that has completed its nourishment-and-repair trip in the feet or other parts of the body below the heart? Amazingly, nature has provided two rather unique ways for blood to travel upward. The first of these is that the veins usually lie between muscles. The other is that they have a built-in system of valves which prevent the blood from flowing backward and keep it on its track toward the heart. If you look at your legs you will notice that the veins seem to weave in among the muscles. Every time a muscle contracts it squeezes a vein; this pushes the blood closer to the heart because the valves prevent the blood from flowing backward. This explains, for instance, why you may suddenly become fatigued or feel sluggish after you have been standing in one position for a long time or sitting down without moving. The blood in the lower part of the body does not get the amount of push it needs from the muscular system and so it does not get back to the heart. This is the cause of varicose veins. The veins begin to lose some of their elastic quality, or the valves in them begin to function improperly, simply because of lack of use. What happens then is that the blood begins to accumulate and this causes the veins to swell.

Up to this point, you undoubtedly will agree that the heart and the circulatory system make up a truly wonderful machine. But this is not all—there are other wonderful things this system accomplishes. For instance, if for some reason the artery or arteries that feed a small area of the bodily tissue—or even a large area—should fail to function, neighboring vessels often take up the burden. From several directions, the tissues that are threatened with a loss of blood supply will receive fresh blood from other arteries that previously did not feed that particular area. In fact, these arteries often grow quite rapidly in size and in length to take over the job of supplying blood. Sometimes they do the job quite as efficiently as the original artery did, and more often than not this action takes place without you yourself ever being aware of the change within your body.

This is vitally necessary because the body is composed of billions of cells and all these cells are nourished by your blood. They are the steadiest of consumers—they demand a constant supply and your ever-faithful heart meets that demand from before you are born until the day that your heart pumps its last "lubb-dub."

The heart, then, is the central engine in a complicated mechanism that is so well devised that it will run smoothly throughout the life of most people. It is so well devised that it always has reserves of power that can be tapped in an emergency. It is so well devised that it can almost always repair itself promptly and effectively. Perhaps the miracle can be brought home more strongly if you try to imagine an automobile running perfectly for seventy years without any more attention than periodic supplies of fuel and water! If you own a car, you look after it with care. Being a normal automobile owner, the moment your car begins to show some signs of wear and tear you take action to repair it. Additionally, you can just go out and buy a new one if it happens to fail to function for its projected lifetime. On the other hand, if your heart fails to perform perfectly after forty or fifty years of neglect, you can't go out and buy a new one. So you panic because your heart has weakened. And it weakened simply because you failed to give it the same attention you would have given your car. You must realize that your heart is very like an engine. It requires—in its own way—at least some of the attention that you lavish on your car.

3

The Causes of Heart Disease

Heart disease kills two persons in the United States every minute. It has become the leading cause of death in men thirty years of age and older in this country. But what is heart disease? And what causes it?

People are always talking about someone who had a "coronary." And you hear such phrases as "cardiac," "heart trouble," "heart failure," "rheumatic heart," "angina," and many other terms—some of them scientific sounding and others no more scientific than "heart attack."

45

Almost everybody can generally recognize most of these terms as relating to a sick heart. But lack of knowledge about this most important of all organs—especially at a time when more than half of all deaths are caused by heart disease—can lead many people to unwarranted fears. On the other hand, it can also lead others to a lack of ordinary precautions that might save their lives.

Studies going on in various countries throughout the world indicate many possible causes for heart disease. Some scientists actually believe that there is a personality type that is prone to heart disease. There are theories that a coronary heart is hereditary, and others that "go-getters" are potential heart victims, that inactivity leads to heart ailments, that anger or fear can bring on a heart attack, that certain kinds of drinking water may be responsible, that viruses may be blamed, and even that nationality and economic strata may make significant differences in the incidence of heart disease.

Heart disease strikes
without warning

The unfortunate thing is that even the most thorough checkup cannot anticipate some defects in the heart. Heart attacks can strike without warning and anyone

46

can be the victim. It is no different than taking your automobile to a garage and having everything checked over. The mechanic may say that the car is in perfect condition and doesn't need anything done to it. But it is possible that there may be a little bit of dirt in the gas tank. Within twenty-four hours that little bit of dirt can be carried into the line that feeds the engine. It can plug the line and gasoline will be unable to get through. The engine will stop. That is exactly what sometimes happens in heart attacks when they occur without warning. Yet there is no way to predict when such a thing will happen. When such a plugging occurs in the bloodstream, the obstruction is known as a thrombus and the stopping of the heart is called coronary thrombosis. This results in what is called myocardial infarction, or destruction of the cells of the heart muscle. That is only one of the major types of heart disease that we know.

The word coronary refers to the arteries which carry the blood into the heart muscle after the blood has been passed into the aorta, the main artery described in the previous chapter. There are two coronary arteries, and they have many branches which reach into every fiber of cardiac muscle. These arteries are the ones that feed oxygen to the heart. The fresh oxygen that the blood gets while it is in the lungs—before being pumped out through the system by the heart—is not touched by the heart in its pumping action. Instead, when the blood is pumped out of the heart, a portion of it is taken off by the coronary arteries and this portion is fed back to the muscles of the heart to feed this muscle tissue in the selfsame way as all the other tissues of the body are fed.

Arterial damage
has many causes

Many factors, including aging, can produce damage in the coronary arteries. This damage is called sclerosis. The most common type is called atherosclerosis. It is as though deposits—something like rust on the inside of a water pipe—clog up in the inner lining of the blood vessels. If these deposits are only in small clusters, they may cause no trouble. But when they get larger and build up one on top of the other so that the passage is narrowed and the blood backs up and clots, then a heart attack occurs. Atherosclerosis is actually a form of arteriosclerosis—and it is probably the most common form. Arteriosclerosis is the general term that is used for all hardening of the arteries which is caused by a thickening of the artery walls or by calcium or fatty deposits. In atherosclerosis, the interior of the artery does not always harden, but the artery wall becomes thick and rough with deposits of a fatty chemical known as cholesterol. The result is clogging.

Actually, there are three major kinds of heart trouble that are caused by atherosclerosis. You have already read a brief description of coronary thrombosis, or coronary occlusion. This occurs when there is a complete blockage—or clotting—of a coronary artery. Such disaster usually causes a myocardial infarction—which, as you have already learned, is the sudden death of great masses of cells in the heart muscle. Pain at the time of such an attack, which does not necessarily come during physical or emotional exertion, is sudden. And it is so severe as to be almost unbearable. It has been described as a vise-like clamp around the chest and it may even extend to the left shoulder, to the neck and the arm. The pain lasts more than a quarter of an hour and may even last for several hours. Accompanying the pain there are irregularities of the heart, difficult breathing, cold sweat, low blood pressure—and sometimes even a fever.

When you hear people talking about "heart attack," they usually mean a coronary occlusion with myocardial infarction.

The second major type of heart trouble caused by atherosclerosis is angina pectoris. In reality, angina pectoris is really more of a symptom, or a warning, of heart disease. What it means is that a spasm of pain has been caused by a momentary inadequacy in the supply of blood reaching the heart muscle. This inadequacy can be caused by a temporary spasm of the artery which will block the flow of blood or it may be caused by a sudden large increase in the heart's demand for blood. This is a condition that is often associated with hypertension, as well as with aging. It is a condition that is more common in men than it is in women.

Pain in an attack of this sort is quite severe—but usually brief. Normally, it will not last for more than a quarter of an hour. It can be brought on by exercise, by an emotional outburst, by overeating, and—more frequently—by worry or fear.

The third major form of heart trouble caused by atherosclerosis is acute coronary insufficiency. This differs from angina pectoris in that in the case of angina the decrease of blood supply is a passing thing. In the case of acute coronary insufficiency, the "starvation" of the heart muscle is much more prolonged. Such an insufficiency occurs usually at times of great physical and emotional stress—times when the demand for blood and oxygen by the heart muscle exceeds the supply. What happens, most often, is that some of the muscle cells die. This condition is most common in men, and particularly in robust, full-blooded men.

What about some of the other diseases that attack the heart? You frequently hear about high blood pressure. In the normal body, various chemicals, as well as the nerves and muscles in the walls of the arteries, work together to keep the pressure of the blood normal. Sudden fright, fear, worry, or tension can make it increase temporarily. In certain people the blood pressure rises slowly over the years. In others, however, the increase is rapid and it continues until it reaches dangerous levels. In a state of hypertension, the increased pressure weakens the arteries and therefore overloads the heart. This causes the heart to become enlarged and highly inefficient. It can also damage other arteries in the body—particularly in the eyes, the kidneys and the brain. High blood pressure increases the chance of a coronary attack and is itself a potentially dangerous disease—one to which, for some reason, women are more susceptible than men.

Coronary arteries
not always involved

Not all heart difficulties, however, are related to the coronary arteries. In fact, there are several totally different categories of disorder to which the heart is subject. Rheumatic fever, for instance, can cause impairment of the heart. If you were to read a list of all the varieties and causes of heart disease, there would probably be more than fifty categories, and that would not include all the subcategories. Let us look at at least some of these other non-coronary causes of heart disease.

The actual cause of rheumatic heart disease is still

unknown. There has in some quarters been suspicion of a streptococcus germ; and even virus infection has been considered. This is a disease that is most common in people under the age of thirty. It is usually accompanied by an attack of rheumatic fever in which numerous joints in the body become swollen, tender and feverish. And while sometimes the attack is accompanied by fever or sore throat, patients are often struck silently when they are young and the damage is not discovered until many years later. In fact, between the ages of fifteen and twenty-five, rheumatic heart disease ranks second to tuberculosis as a cause of death. This disease may attack any part of the heart, but usually the main heart valves are affected and you will often hear of people referring to "leaky" valves due to such an attack.

In some instances where a person has an extremely low metabolism due to underactivity of the thyroid gland—known as myxedema—the heart may become enlarged and show evidence of failure. At the other extreme it is overactivity of the thyroid gland—called increased metabolism—in which there is a disturbance of the heart's function called auricular fibrillation.

A person can often be stricken with syphilitic heart disease following an infection with syphilis. This may lie dormant for fifteen or twenty years after the original infection and then suddenly become full-blown.

Endocarditis is a form of heart infection in which germs attack the lining of the heart valves. There are

52

more than half a dozen different forms of endocarditis.

Congenital heart disease is a defect acquired before birth and is due to malformation in the heart. This is the medical term for what are better known as "blue babies."

Nervous heart and functional heart diseases are conditions in which the patient presents many symptoms which resemble organic heart disease, yet after careful study no disease can be found.

You can live

after heart failure

The purpose for listing all these—and there are countless others—is that should you ever be told that you have "heart disease," you should realize that you cannot compare yourself with your uncle who collapsed several years ago, or with anyone else who suffered from "heart disease." It is important that you bear in mind that there is a distinction between the various types of heart disease.

People often wonder why some patients still live after having had a "heart failure." This is probably because these patients have had what is known as a congestive heart failure—a term that is rather misleading since it does not always mean that the heart stops beating.

This is a condition which can accompany and complicate any type of heart disease simply because at the moment of the attack the heart fails as a pump to keep the circulation going at a satisfactory pace. Throughout the body, there is built up what might be termed an "oxygen debt" when not enough blood is circulated. If this debt cannot be repaid by increasing the heartbeat or the amount of blood circulated with each heartbeat, then the heart is also being starved for oxygen and heart failure occurs. Chronic congestive heart failure can afflict people who live under great daily stress and whose demands for blood and oxygen are, therefore, too great for the heart's pumping power. A sudden extra demand can mean complete heart failure and death.

For more than a decade the American Heart Association has been helping thousands of medical researchers in their work of trying to pinpoint the causes of strain, and eventual disintegration, of the heart muscle. And while the reasons seem to be spread through a score or more fields, little by little the finger seems to be pointing more and more to one major cause—*stress*. More precisely, the answer seems to lie in the individual's reaction to stress.

III

You and Stress

4

What Is Stress?

Stress is the body's reaction to wear and tear. Every single activity, every emotion—whether it's crossing a busy street, whether it's exposing yourself to a draft, whether it's kissing someone—each sets up a stress. It is believed that most diseases, perhaps even all diseases, stem from this common cause. And it is believed that in the body's reaction to stress, governed largely by inherited physical characteristics, lies the secret of good health and longevity.

It was just about a quarter-century ago that a young

Austrian endocrinologist published a brief medical paper which outlined what he called a "stress syndrome." From that tiny seed has grown a huge new concept of disease, a concept that has been called the greatest single contribution to the realm of biology and medicine since Louis Pasteur. The man responsible is Hans Selye. The man himself, aside from his work, is so fascinating that it would take an entire book to tell you about him. But his work, and the countless thousands of experiments it has keyed, now fill many shelves in every medical library the world over.

One of the great advances of modern medicine was the increasing recognition of the importance of emotions in influencing bodily health. This is the view that recognizes that both the mind and the body work together as one and that the mind reacts upon the body as well as the body reacting upon the mind. This knowledge that all illnesses must be considered and treated in relation to the entire person forms the foundation for psychosomatic medicine. The word psychosomatic comes from two Latin terms: *psyche,* meaning the mind, and *soma,* meaning the body. Although this term was first used in medicine in Germany more than a hundred years ago, it did not come into common use until the great Dr. Flanders Dunbar introduced it into medicine on this continent at just about the same time that Dr. Selye introduced to the medical world his theory of the stress syndrome. And while today the theory of stress has created new highways along which medical research must inevitably travel, it is a concept which has perhaps long dwelled in man's unconscious mind.

Robert Louis Stevenson, for instance, once wrote:

> Look at one of your industrious fellows. He sows hurry and reaps indigestion; he puts a vast deal of activity out to interest and receives a large measure of nervous derangement in return.

Perhaps if we were to say the same thing today we might state it as: Stress will get you if you don't watch out!

*An essential
factor of life*

Stress is not the villain that some magazine articles make it out to be. Dr. Selye makes it very clear that stress is not necessarily harmful. The trouble arises, however, when stress is unduly prolonged or when it comes too often or when it is concentrated on one particular organ of the body. What stress does is set off some of the body's glands so that they spurt hormone substances into your system which enable your body to deal with a particular situation in an appropriate manner. The agent that creates the stress is called the "stressor." For example, if you are in the African wilds and a lion suddenly charges at you, this stressor will set off your adrenal glands, which in turn will force adrenalin into your system. The adrenalin is necessary to make you have the necessary physical and mental responses—responses that will either get you out of there as quickly as possible or have you pick up your rifle and attempt to kill the beast. When the excitement is over, other hormones will be released by other glands which will enable your body to quickly revert to normal activity. A stressor, however, need not be such a violent one. It can be a soft hand stroking your forehead, and hormonal changes enable you to deal with this just as they help you deal with a lion. When the soft, stroking hand stressor is the catalytic agent, you may become amorous —or perhaps you may drop off into a restful sleep.

While chemical changes resulting from stress play a more destructive part in life than had been believed up to now, Dr. Selye insists that some stress may well be a vital factor in life. In fact, he feels it is often the spice of life since any emotion or any activity can cause it. Nor, of course, should stress be thought of as purely a matter of simple addition. That is to say, it is not like the last straw that breaks the proverbial camel's back. It is, rather, precipitated by the interaction of the accumulated "straws." And this interaction determines the rate of wear and tear about which Dr. Selye talks.

Stress starts
at childbirth

Without some stress you would not be alive. A mother in childbirth and the baby being born are both under stress. The baby straining to sit up for the first time or tensely balancing to take its first steps is under stress. The athlete striving to win a race, the artist trying to produce his best work, the man trying to double as father and mother to his family while his wife is sick —all these are under stress. The patient struggling feverishly to regain health is just as much under stress as the doctor who is treating him. The workingman, attempting to do his job to the best of his ability, is just as much under stress as his employer, who worries continually about business problems both at the office and at home. The truth of the matter is that nobody can escape stress. The varying degrees and the different forms of stress all have some impact. That impact can sometimes be good, and sometimes harmful. It may have damaging side effects which can lead to disease, can cause aging prematurely, or can even shorten life.

Since all normal living causes wear and tear on the

body, the only measurement possible of that wear and tear is stress. But the body, under normal circumstances, repairs the wear and tear. As body cells are worn out, they are replaced with new ones. And by this action of replacement, the body grows and strengthens itself. It is logical, then, that some stress is good for you under certain circumstances. The vital factor is that stress itself is not the great danger, but it is the effects of stress that are.

Although you are constantly under strains of various kinds which keep you continually in a state of tension, you do not necessarily show stress symptoms because your mind and your body are working together to make the necessary, often automatic, adjustments. You breathe more deeply to replenish oxygen when it is needed. You sleep when you are tired. You eat when you are hungry. It is only where the strains imposed are excessive, or unexpected, or prolonged that serious symptoms of stress actually appear. If you should swallow a dose of poison for which there is no antidote, the strain is excessive. If you are struck a blow in the face, and are completely unprepared for it, the strain is unexpected. If you overwork yourself continuously, the strain is prolonged.

Though stress is not easy to define because it is something which we are only aware of through its effects, it is, nonetheless, quite different from strain and from tension. To take a simple example, so that you can differentiate between the three terms, imagine two big, burly tug-of-war teams. They stand facing each other, with the heavy rope stretched between them and ready. At the word "go," they try to pull each other over the line. Just before they start to heave, they experience the strain. When the signal to begin is given, the rope is pulled sharply from both ends and it is in a state of tension. The effect of this tension upon the rope—that is, the wear and tear that develops during this tug-of-war—is the symptom of stress.

The trail that
led to stress

A question that bothered Dr. Selye when he was still a young medical student in Europe led him to his eventual discovery. His professors always talked about specific diseases with specific causes. But young Selye kept wondering about non-specific diseases—about the feeling of "just being sick." His professors had little patience with this nonsense, as they termed it. But this didn't bother the young Austrian student. After years of following false trails he came upon the discovery, almost by chance, that stress produced symptoms in his experimental animals which in turn caused decay and death. From this he evolved his theory of the "general adaptation syndrome"—abbreviated to G-A-S, and also called the "stress syndrome." It comprises three stages:

First, there is an *alarm*. It is the body's response to any stressor agent, such as infectious organisms, chemicals, hormones, cold, heat, radiation, trauma, pain. It is like a call to arms, a partial or general mobilization of the body's defenses when an invader threatens.

Second, there is *resistance*. Certain glands in the body begin to produce hormones which come to grips with the invader and either repel it or seek to establish an acceptable way of adapting to it so that it can give no further trouble.

Finally, there is *exhaustion*. This occurs when stress is prolonged and the body's mechanism, trying to adapt to the stress, breaks down. The result is a loss of resistance. No living organism can be kept permanently at the "alarm" stage. If the exposure is too long, or if the enemies are too powerful, the ability of the body to resist and to adapt is lost. The result is, obviously, death —something which life eventually imposes upon everyone.

The secret of health, therefore, lies in the successful adjustment to changing stresses. The penalty for failure in this great process of adaptation is ill health and, naturally, unhappiness. Although you cannot avoid stresses as long as you live, you can learn how to keep their damaging side effects to a minimum. In this sense,

64

many nervous and emotional disturbances which appear to be essentially diseases of adaptation can, perhaps, be controlled. And among these disturbances can be listed diseases of the heart.

Since stress is not always damaging, it is important that you realize why stress is not necessarily bad for you. The point is, stress can be a plus-factor in living just as long as your system is prepared to take it. The same stress which makes one person sick can be an invigorating experience for another person. As Dr. Selye has pointed out, no one can live without experiencing some degree of stress all the time. You may think that only serious diseases or intensive mental or physical injury can cause stress. This, however, is false. Every bit of living entails stress. You cannot avoid it as long as you live.

Stress and

cardiac failure

Since the heart is the most vital organ of the body, it is natural that Dr. Selye's experimentation should have led him to investigate the results of stress as they affect the heart. With his staff of researchers at the modern buildings at the University of Montreal, Dr. Selye began to give special attention to cardiac failures. Rats and other animals whose hormone balance had been purposely upset were found to suffer heart lesions when subjected to stress. Various forms of stress were developed so that the animals could be tested. Some were taped firmly to boards. Some were made to swim for several minutes in cold water. Others were placed in refrigerators and then quickly warmed up in hot chambers. Some were made to run for hours at a time in motor-driven revolving cages.

Dr. Selye found that healthy animals could take such treatment in their stride, but those whose hormones had been upset in some fashion quickly succumbed. If sodium salts had been given to the animals the end was even quicker. But these results were not really new. Dr. Selye and his assistants had known for some time that animals could be given heart lesions if their hormones were tampered with and if the animals were then exposed to intense stress. These experiments merely confirmed the theory that Dr. Selye had that stress of mind and body can deliver the fatal blow when other upsets, such as a hormone imbalance, pave the way.

But the important discovery was that serious heart disease was found in all the animals which were given the stress tests—except those which had had doses of potassium and magnesium. Having noticed that sodium salts had speeded up the heart damage, Dr. Selye had attempted to counteract this salt by giving some of the animals the other two salts. The potassium and mag-

66

nesium not only worked against the sodium, they saved the animals. The changes that appeared in these animals parallel those that appear in adult humans who have lived through years of stress. And the results are encouraging since it seems possible that by determining the chemical reaction of the body to stress, it may eventually be possible to find a way of counteracting—chemically—this fatal reaction.

5

Why You Get Keyed Up

Every one of you is familiar with the feeling of being keyed up from nervous tension. This process is quite comparable to raising the pitch of a violin string by tightening it. You certainly must admit that your muscles will limber up during exercise and that you will be thrilled by great emotional experiences. All of this toning up prepares you for better peak accomplishments. On the other hand, there is jitteriness when you are too keyed up. This impairs your work and even prevents you from getting a rest.

Being keyed up is a true sensation, but it has its basis in a physiochemical reaction. This reaction has not yet been fully analyzed, but science does know that at the time of tension your adrenal glands produce an excess of adrenalins (which stimulate the heart) and of corticoids. For example, a person who has been given a large dose of cortisone in order to treat some allergy or perhaps a rheumatic condition may find it difficult to sleep. As a matter of fact, he may even become abnormally keyed up—carried away by an unreasonable sense of well-being and buoyancy which is not unlike the sensation of being slightly drunk. However, a sense of deep depression may follow this. It has long been known that not only mental excitements—such as excitements communicated by a rioting mob or by some act of violence—but even physical stressors, such as a burn, can cause an initial excitement which is followed by depression later on. Experiments by Dr. Selye's researchers showed that there were definitely identifiable chemical compounds that were produced by the body's hormones during the acute "alarm" reaction phase of G-A-S. These compounds were found to possess the property of first keying you up for action and then causing a depression. Dr. Selye says that both these effects may be of great practical value to your body. It is obviously necessary to be keyed up so that you can have big accomplishments. But it is equally important to be tuned down in that secondary phase of depression, since this is the check valve that prevents you from pushing on for too great a length of time at top speed.

Stress hormone
intoxication

Stress, it appears, can stimulate your glands to produce hormones. Hormones, in turn, can induce a kind of drunkenness. Without knowing this, however, you would never think of checking your conduct as carefully during stress as you do at a cocktail party. Yet, you should. The fact is, Dr. Selye states, that you can be intoxicated with your own stress hormones. This sort of drunkenness may have caused much more harm to society than the other kind. The difficulty is, you are constantly on guard against external intoxicants. However, hormones are definite and distinct parts of the body— and it takes more wisdom to recognize and overcome a foe which fights from within. In every action throughout the day you must consciously look for signs of being keyed up too much, and you must learn to stop in time. Watching your critical stress-level is just as important as watching your critical quota of cocktails. In fact, it seems likely that it is even more important. Intoxication by stress is sometimes unavoidable and is usually quite insidious. You can stop taking alcohol; and even if you do take some, you can at least count how much you have had. In the same way, you ought to be able to keep track of your stress-alarm signals.

Unfortunately, the pituitary gland is often a better judge of stress than the intellect is. Any time there is an emergency, the body is prepared for this emergency through the pituitary hormone known as ACTH. This hormone has achieved its greatest fame through its use in arthritis treatment.

What happens is this: Any time there is an "attack" on the body, an SOS is sent out to warn of the attack. This attack may be an invasion by disease germs, it may be an emotional crisis, or it may be an injury. Let us say that it is an injury. The injury sets off an "alarm" reaction within the body. The nervous system sends out the first danger signal, and among the defense forces first activated are hormones which are quickly sent into action. With the aid of these chemicals, the body gets ready to handle the emergency. The pituitary gland, a tiny thing located under the brain, dispatches ACTH. This special hormone signals the adrenal glands, which are just above the kidneys. In turn, the adrenal glands send out other hormones which do their share to help heal the injury.

These two glands balance the body's chemistry so that disease can be resisted or injury can be healed without overly disturbing the working order of the rest of the system.

71

As has been pointed out previously, however, strong emotions can be just as responsible for these bodily changes. For example, fear will make you tense. And when fear occurs, hormones speed through your system and cause your heart to beat rapidly. The muscles of your stomach and intestines contract and force your blood into quick circulation. Your breathing increases and a number of other changes occur which help to bring you to a point at which you can meet the emergency or pass through the difficult situation.

You cannot recognize
destructive stresses

There is no doubt that normal emotional stress can be useful in many ways. You may get very excited about a job that is interesting and important and, as a result, you will be able to handle the work with greater efficiency and effectiveness. There are emotions that are quite pleasurable—and these involve stresses and tensions that can bring exhilaration. Perhaps you get excited and tense while watching a baseball game or a boxing match. This type of tension can give you a great deal of pep. And the letdown that follows is, in fact, healthy relaxation. It is important, therefore, to know that the emotional stress that you are aware of is usually stress that is good for you—not bad for you. If it were not for this stress, you would be living more or less like a vegetable, without any feeling.

The stress, however, that is destructive is the kind that you don't recognize. It is the stress that comes from intense persistent anger, the stress that comes from fear and frustration, the stress that comes from worry. These are stresses that you may bottle up inside yourself. These are the stresses that can threaten your health. It is these undue emotional stresses that lead to trouble; it is not the emotions themselves.

The relationship
between stress and disease

Recent studies have shown that perhaps more than half the people who seek medical aid are suffering from illnesses which have been brought about, or worsened, by prolonged stress. Even the simplest organic illness can be developed into a serious condition by too much worry, or too much anxiety, or too much fear. When tension of this type is too often repeated, or when it continues for a long time, then the chemistry of your body reaches the point of imbalance. This imbalance develops any time you overwork to excess, or worry to the point where you cannot take it easy, or are under such pressure that you can no longer get a good night's sleep.

A recent study in New York City highlighted the dangerous relationship between stress and disease. The doctors who conducted this study selected a group of more than one thousand women who were about the same age, who had the same training and income, and who were employed under similar conditions by one large company. They discovered that close to one-third of these women were responsible for four times as much time lost due to sickness as the rest of the group. In studying this group of sick women, they found that they were generally women who had more responsibilities and worries, women who had a great deal of extra hard work and frustrations. It turned out that many of them were widows and divorcées who had small children to care for. They were struggling through a life of disappointments and insecurity. A similar study was also made of a group of men employed by a large company under similar working conditions and opportunities. Again they found that about one-third of the men were responsible for more than seventy-five per cent of all the illness. These men were also under pressure from their life situations. Interviews showed that some felt they had been trapped by economic pressures in their jobs. Others indicated that their wives were ill or that they had too many children to look after. Some told of unhappy marriages that were continually marred by arguments. Others of the group were ambitious but were frustrated by a lack of advancement.

Interestingly enough, among the groups of men and women who were sick, a variety of illnesses were reported. But a high percentage showed distinct problems of high blood pressure leading to heart failure.

A more recent study found that the hard-driving career woman has in common with her male counterpart a higher-than-average incidence of heart disease. This study found that career women had five to eight times as much heart disease as housewives or other career women who were not as hard-driving. The results were interesting in that they disproved an earlier theory that had indicated that women executives were less prone to heart disease than their male counterparts. But we do not have to limit the taxing tensions to executives, either male or female. The average woman is taxed by tensions every day. Recent studies showed that the average mother of three children has a weekly workload that includes washing more than 700 dishes and more than 400 pieces of cutlery; handling some 250 pieces of laundry; making beds 35 times; shopping for, carrying, and cooking 175 pounds of food; and walking between 30 and 35 miles while doing housework. And the average housewife and mother has little chance for escaping the crises that occur in her home.

It seems that no one—workman or housewife, executive or educator, professional or career woman—no

75

one can escape the tensions that tax the body in every insidious way possible.

Coping with stress in daily living

While nobody underestimates the job of being a housewife and a mother, it has been found that men especially seem to have ailments which can most often be traced to prolonged tension. It seems that in spite of the many responsibilities involved, a woman's work at home apparently does not entail the same type of strain which most men undergo from day to day while working.

Is it that men are weaker than women? Or is it that men usually have to cope with more stress in their daily lives than women? It seems that men often drive themselves beyond their endurance because so much seems to be expected of them. Many try to live up to a picture of masculinity which portrays them as being superhuman individuals, men who can take it, who can live and work and play without any signs of weakness. It seems that being the breadwinner—whether man or woman— is a difficult job. Tension is inevitable. The job of homemaker, on the other hand, gives the woman some time— if she desires it—to relax and let some things go. She can often find time for interesting hobbies right at home. She can vary her activities. She can usually take time to rest during the day. This is not so with the bread-winner. The family's livelihood and security hinge on the way the breadwinner handles his job. He is often faced with competition for a job or for advances in his position. Just the realization of the responsibility is enough to make many men feel tense and anxious at all times.

Medicine has based its knowledge that emotions play an important part in many kinds of physical illnesses on facts with which you are all familiar. In everyday situations everyone has experienced some of the effects of emotions. Certainly you have blushed at some time or another. Or you have had a tight feeling in your chest or a weight in the pit of your stomach before some important event. You have felt your heart pound and seen your hands perspire when you have been excited or afraid. These are normal reactions to specific situations. They are beyond your control. They are reactions which usually disappear quickly once the cause of them has been removed. These changes occur simply because emotion is meant to make you act. Fear will make you tense. And the heart will beat more rapidly. Rapid heartbeat is a familiar part of many emotions, however. In some people, when the emotional tension is pro-longed, heart palpitation may occur so readily that the person suffering from it may no longer be aware of the

77

emotion that originally started it. This person then becomes filled with new fears, worrying about whether his symptoms mean that he has a serious disease. Worry can influence the severity and duration of any illness.

"Body language" of emotionally induced diseases

An emotional conflict which you may suffer is sometimes so difficult for you to accept that you may repress your feelings altogether. You become completely unconscious of the fact that they exist. Often what seems to be a physical illness stems from a hidden wish to accomplish an end quite different from the one obviously demanded by the situation, and one which you are not aware of. There are many examples of the unconscious mind's protest against doing something that you do not want to do. Perhaps you have developed a headache just before having to attend an unwelcome appointment. Your protest caused your head to ache in the hope that perhaps you would not have to go because of the organic illness that developed. Physical distress can often be a kind of body language to express emotional troubles that have been repressed. Some of the most common expressions in the language show that we all use some of this body language of the emotions.

78

There are countless examples, such as "pain in the neck," "oh, my aching back," "I am fed up to here," "he burns me up," "my blood ran cold," "more than I can stomach," "a lump in my throat." Everyone has had some emotionally induced illness at some time or another. The late Dr. John Schindler made a short list of symptoms that could be induced emotionally and indicated in terms of percentages just how often the occurrence of each was due to emotions. His list included such complaints as: "gas," more than 99% of the time; "lump in the throat" and "tiredness," 90% of the time; "headaches" and "dizziness," 80% of the time; and "pain in the back of the neck," 75% of the time.

Every time, therefore, that something "threatens" you, there is an emotional reaction—a reaction of tension and stress. The threat can be anything: difficulty at home, opposition at work, fear of failure. The list could probably go on and on for pages and pages. What happens inside you when you experience tension is very much like what happens at a firehouse when an alarm is sounded. Before the alarm rings, the firemen are sitting around going about their normal routine. Everything is calm and pleasant. The situation is the equivalent of a state of equilibrium with you. Then suddenly the alarm rings. The stressor is made known to you. There is a sharp transformation instantly. In the fire station the men race to their posts. Everything is in a keyed-up state as all equipment gets ready to fight the "enemy." Soon the firemen and their engines are racing to the scene of the trouble. They go into action to attack the enemy and destroy it. Once the fire is out, the return to equilibrium begins—the pace begins to slow, the action subsides, and the tension eases. When the equilibrium is restored, the tension is gone. Your whole system reacts in the selfsame way.

The only way to fight the tension is to overcome it— to learn to relax and to bring back your equilibrium.

6

How to Tune Down

While anxiety and tension are essential functions of living—just as are hunger and thirst—there is a time when you have to become watchful so that they do not overwhelm you.

If you had no tensions, how could you ever stand up for your rights? How could you ever dodge a speeding car while crossing the street? But if you have too much tension, you suddenly find that the juice has been squeezed out of comfortable living. Too much tension takes the bounce out of your life; it causes you to race your motor and to run so fast that you never see the landscape around you, only the mileposts as you pass.

The difficulty is that too many people look upon life as the Norsemen of old did upon Heaven. To them, Heaven was a time to be passed in daily battles, with all of their wounds magically healed. What a wonderful myth—but only a myth. Every one of you has to meet demands on your nervous energy, demands that were not made in former years. The farmer who was once looked upon as living the most tranquil life now has to face many economic, social and political problems, problems of which his grandfather was ignorant. The lawyer and the doctor both have clients pressing at their office doors—and they are conscious that others need them at all times and in other places. Teachers have the unenviable task of maintaining discipline in a brood more restless than ever before. Stenographers are typing many words a minute; factory workers are engaged in countless operations; tellers in the bank try to meet the wants of customers with flawless accuracy.

Every one of you is working under conditions that strain the physical, the mental, and the emotional structure built during ages of evolution. Nor is your immediate environment all that counts. From radio news reports that you listen to at the breakfast table to the late news on television before bedtime—not to count the newspaper you read during the day—you are under the pressure of battling within yourself world difficulties. You are constantly exposed to tension, constantly expecting some new crisis.

Learn to recognize

tension-makers

The tensions you live with are sometimes hard to recognize. You call them by other names: bills past due, unfairness, in-laws, deadlines. You call them anything that causes you to tighten up inside. So when someone says, "You ought to stop getting keyed up and start getting tuned down!"—and says it again and again— you probably get exasperated. After all, how do you tune down?

The first thing you must do is recognize your tensions for what they are. Next you have to apply simple and practical measures to help yourself relax, measures that have helped other people in a practical fashion to do the same thing. You will then discover how completely different it feels to be relaxed than it does to be tense— not only completely different, but so blissful. The unfortunate thing is that there is no panacea. There is no magic formula nor pill you can take that will guarantee you an overnight cure. If you are overly tense, you have undoubtedly been living with tensions for a long time. And once you have lived with something for a long time, it is going to take perhaps a great deal of time—and patience—to soothe those tensions and to gentle them. So before you start to tune down, you must remember a simple three-word formula: *Easy does it!*

Your ability to relax is one of the surest symptoms of your mental health. After you have been keyed up to accomplish a task, you need to slacken off instead of whipping yourself into new exertion. If you relax away the little tensions as they occur, you stand a very good chance of preventing the accumulation of big tensions. These small relaxations are simple. For every tension-making situation, there is a relaxation-making counteraction.

How often have you found minor problems and small disappointments throwing you into a dither? Or do you find getting along with people difficult more and more often? Have you found that the small pleasures of life no longer satisfy you? Or are you unable to stop thinking of your anxieties? Do people or situations that never used to bother you before now cause you a great deal of apprehension? Have you become suspicious of people in general, and mistrustful of your friends? Answering yes to these questions does not necessarily mean disaster. But it does indicate that you are no different from the rest of the population. It indicates that you need to deal with situations of this sort.

84

The physical
causes of tension

Tensions wind you up and leave you with no place to go. Picture yourself as a sprinter. You are crouched at the starting line and the starter has called, "*On your mark . . . get set . . .*" But he never fires the starting gun. There you are. Your muscles are quivering to push your body forward and dash to the finish line. You get wound up more and more tightly, your eyes begin to bug out, your teeth clench and grit. That's exactly what all your tensions do to you. People who are not relaxed, who are overtense, usually have increased muscle tone. However, it is so imperceptible that they usually are not aware of it. How capable are you of controlling your muscles? Can you make them go limp? Think of the muscles in your shoulders and in your neck. Let them go limp. That wasn't hard, was it? But until you relaxed those muscles *consciously*, you actually were not aware that there were feelings of tension in the muscles.

The big problem is, of course, that muscles have no initiative. They never tighten nor do they relax except when they are commanded to. The commands arrive over the "telegraph" of the nervous system. The nerves tell the muscles to get tense and get ready to run the race, but the race never starts. The muscles cannot judge whether or not the order is reasonable.

85

The race, however, doesn't have to be a physical one. It can be a mental one. It can be the anxiety of trying to get a promotion over the man who is working beside you. It is situations of this sort that can frighten you, can anger you, can worry or depress or discourage you. It is situations of this sort against which, however, you do not—and perhaps cannot—take direct effective action.

Mental tension and muscle tension go together. You cannot have one without the other. So before going on to mental tensions and how you can relax them, you should understand something about muscle tensions. There is an old story about a man who banged his head against the wall simply because it felt good when he stopped. Perhaps you can still laugh at that silly story— but maybe it isn't as silly as you think. Try "making a muscle" in your upper arm, extending your arm and bending it with a clenched fist. Tighten every muscle in your arm as hard as you can and try to hold your arm steady. It won't be long before your fist will be quivering with a fine flutter. Now, relax your hand completely. Open the fingers and let the arm go limp. Your hand will be steady as a steamroller. That is the quiet strength of relaxation.

That little experiment should help you recognize your muscle tensions consciously so that in the future you can recognize them almost automatically. Try wrinkling your brow and then relaxing it. Hunch up your shoulders and then relax them. Pull in your stomach tightly, and then relax. Every time you relax—and the tension goes—you feel better. The sooner you can learn how to do this consciously every time there is physical tension, the sooner you will train yourself to respond that way unconsciously. And once you learn the secret of unconsciously loosening your muscles, you will be on the road to making a habit of relaxation.

Learning to relax
your muscles

Now the important thing is to recognize in yourself the areas that cause you the most muscle-tension problems. There are several groups of muscles that are favorite sites of high-tension trouble. Among these are the abdomen, the shoulders, the face and neck, the hands and arms, and even the legs. Keep an eye on yourself, and keep your nervous system alert for aches and pains that may tip you off to muscle tensions. Do you tighten your lips or clamp your jaw? Do you grit your teeth or maybe furrow your brow? Do the muscles in your neck and back tense up? Do you find yourself sitting stiffly at the edge of your chair, or leaning tensely over your desk? Do you hold on to things with almost a death-grip—such as a pencil when you write, or the steering wheel of your car when you're driving? These are the little clues that may point to high-tension trouble.

When you want to, it is very simple to relax a muscle. You can slump into an easy chair without any elaborate instructions. The trick is, however, discovering how to relax consciously so that once you have figured out how you do it, you can continue to do so unconsciously—and habitually. There are many small relaxations that you can practice. Do you commute to work? Then why not close your eyes on the train or bus? Do you find people constantly telling you their troubles? Why not try slackening your muscles while you are listening? Try changing your pace occasionally—sometimes walk leisurely from the office to the bus stop, other times walk briskly.

If you find your jaws and lips and neck muscles tightening every so often, try yawning. Open wide with a real big yawn, wag your jaw a little bit and chew on air with your mouth open. This is a favorite exercise for vocal students since it gives them more flexible jaws and throat muscles.

At a free moment behind your desk, try just slumping to relax your position. Bend and twist the kinks out. You can do this whether you are sitting or standing. Let your hands flop from your wrists—but quite vigorously. Let the fingers fly any which way. The funny feeling you will have is the joints easing up and untensing, and your circulation being speeded through the circulatory system. When you find your leg and back muscles tightening up after a hard day sitting behind your desk, stretch hard. Roll your shoulders and swing your arms as you would trying to keep warm on a cold and windy plain. Do a little shadow-boxing. You will be surprised how much tension it will take out of you.

At least once a day take a few minutes to stretch out upon your bed, flat on your back. Prop up your knees and your neck—and any other parts of your body that are tense—with pillows. You'll soon learn where the pillows feel best. Then let the muscles all through your body go limp one by one. Start at the very bottom of your feet. Relax your toes and slowly work your way up the body until the tiniest muscle on the top of your scalp is relaxed. If your muscles are perfectly relaxed you will never know it, because by that time you will be dozing.

Emotions make

tensions, too!

What about your emotional tensions? Why not take a look at a few of the most common ones? Worry probably ranks number one with everyone. The easiest way to see your own worry in a clearer light is to try talking things out with someone you can trust. Confide your worry to a level-headed person; do not bottle it up.

89

You may select a member of your family or perhaps your religious adviser, or it may be your family doctor. It should be anyone to whom you feel you can talk in confidence. You will be surprised how talking things out helps you to relieve your strain and often helps you to see what you can do about the cause of your worry.

What about anger? Do you let anger get the better of you, or do you try working it out of your system so that you are better prepared to handle the problem that caused the anger in the first place? If you find yourself using anger as a general pattern of behavior, remember that anger will generally leave you feeling foolish and sorry after it is all over. If you really feel like lashing out at someone, try not only counting ten—keep counting for twenty-four hours. In other words, this is one instance where you should put off until tomorrow what you would rather do today. And in the meantime, use up the energy you have in physical activity. Get on the golf course and play eighteen holes; go down into your workshop and fix the table that your wife has been pestering you about for months; go into the kitchen and whip up a cake for dinner. Once you get the anger out of your system in this way, you will be surprised how much easier it is to cope with the irritant.

When a problem becomes too painful, why not follow the same advice as you might to cope with anger— put it off until later rather than face the situation now. Sometimes it helps to escape from a painful problem for a short while. If you try to make yourself stand there and suffer, you are only punishing yourself more. And that is hardly the way to solve any problem. Pick up a book and read for a while, go to a movie, take a walk, go out to the ball park. Any change of scene will do the trick—provided, however, that you are prepared to come back and deal with the difficulty when you are more composed and in a better condition to deal with it, both emotionally and intellectually.

One of the biggest causes of the high-tension terrors is frustration in dealing with other people. There is no real need to always be right, especially if you find yourself getting into frequent quarrels with other people. All that happens is you begin to feel obstinate and defiant. But remember, that is the way children feel and behave. After all, there is always the possibility that you could be wrong in any particular situation. But even if you are completely right, it is far easier on your system to give in once in a while. And if you do this, you will usually find that other people will give in, too. The overall result is going to be quick relief from high-tension terrors.

And what about the work load that seems so big that it either intimidates you or brings out the superman urge within you to try it all at once? To most people who are suffering from high-tension terrors, an ordinary work load looks so great that it seems painful to tackle even some small part of it. The best thing to do in such a situation is to pick the most urgent part of the work load and tackle that. Set aside the others for the time being. Then, once you have disposed of the urgent matter, see if the rest does not go easier—just as long as you take one thing at a time. On the other hand, don't build your tension level to the point of exhaustion by feeling that you haven't achieved all you could. There is no need to achieve perfection in everything. This is a wonderful ideal, but it's a direct invitation to failure. Decide the thing that you can do best, then do it the best you can. The other tasks should be done to the best of your ability, but you should not build up your frustration if you find that you cannot achieve perfection in them as you did in your forte.

Exasperation and frustration:
public enemies

Above all, try a little bit of the new anti-tension drug: *Consideration*. If you are worrying about yourself all the time, try doing something for someone else. Try not expecting too much from other people—whether it is your co-worker in business, an employee, your boss, your husband, your wife, or even one of your children. Remember that everyone should develop on his own and not in any set pattern that *you* think suits him best.

92

Instead of being critical of other people, try to help them by searching out their best points and aiding in the development of these. Don't go around competing with everyone in life—try cooperating. This is just as important in the office or the home as it is on the highway. Every time you try to race somebody, there is a strong likelihood that someone is going to end up injured. Try giving other people a break, and you will be surprised how much easier it makes things for you. Make yourself available for other people; it will take the steam out of your worries and will give you a warm feeling, a deep satisfaction in the knowledge that you have done well for someone else and helped to gain some perspective on yourself.

There are all kinds of exasperations every day that get you keyed up. While modern invention and labor-saving machinery have relieved much of the physical drudgery of day-to-day living, there are definite signs that they have increased nervous strain. Aided by all your gadgets, you live at high speed. You always meet deadlines, you always chase to catch a train, you always grab a bite to eat on the run. Your toes are tramped on and your temper is frayed as you fight to get aboard the home-bound bus. The tension of work accompanies you home, it keeps you awake—unless you have worked out for yourself an effective way of releasing it. One of the evil results of hasty living is that so often you fail to solve your problems adequately. Much of the time you are tangled up in the woolly words with which you clothe your thoughts rather than the facts themselves. The result is a state of high-tension terror.

You have found in earlier chapters that it is wholesome to have fear when that fear is an alarm bell, a warning of impending danger. The difficulty is, however, that too many people go around in a perpetual state of anxiety, almost as though they still think that the world is flat and that they may fall over the edge. This anxiety prevents you from relaxing. This anxiety keeps you tense. And the protective patterns that are set in motion by your body are overworked.

All of this is not to say, of course, that everyone should not fight for whatever seems really worthwhile to him. On the other hand, you should aim only for things that are attainable; otherwise frustration is sure to set in. Although he has written hundreds of thousands of words to support and explain his theories of stress, Dr. Selye has come up with a simple fourteen-word motto that you should keep with you at all times in your efforts to tune down. This motto is:

> Fight always for the highest attainable aim,
> But never put up resistance in vain.

It may take you a little time to learn how to fill that prescription correctly, but it will be well worth the effort.

7

The Importance of Sleep

One of the greatest drains on man's emotional and physical reserve is lack of sleep. Sleeplessness is a symptom common to most illnesses. And the lack of sleep, bringing on fatigue in turn, can actually cause heart symptoms in the absence of real heart disease. Indeed, sleeplessness is becoming a major national problem. A recent survey showed that more than half the adults in the United States are chronic non-sleepers. And, as a result, one of the biggest booms in business has been in the area of sleeping pills and mechanical sleep-inducers. It

95

has been estimated that well over five hundred tons of sleeping pills are sold to Americans every year. And a myriad of sleep-inducing gadgets are on the market—all of them selling well. There are eye shades, ear plugs, mattress pulsators, muscle massagers, and more than you can shake a foam rubber pillow at.

Almost any healthy person you speak to will point out how important he or she finds sleep. And not just "sufficient sleep," but "plenty of sleep." By plenty of sleep these people mean that they sleep long enough and frequently enough to awaken feeling well rested. If you are not well rested or if you do not get sufficient sleep, you cannot enjoy the best of health. Only through sleep do your muscles—and, more important, your nervous system—get a chance to replenish themselves to the fullest. Sleep is virtually the most important way you can find to prevent your machinery from running down.

It is probably not an exaggeration to say that millions of people take their sleeping habits far too lightly. What you may fail to realize is that between the ages of twenty and seventy you are likely to spend more than fifteen full years in bed. In that fifty-year period, you are likely to fall asleep close to twenty thousand separate times. And yet, despite the fact that in your adult years you may spend approximately one-third of your life sleeping, the chances are that you are not getting the most out of your sleep.

Estimate your own
sleep requirements

Just as you have to find out what your own particular
needs are in the way of relaxation, so you must estimate
accurately your own needs in the way of sleep. Your
sleep requirements may range from one or two hours
a day to twelve hours a day. But you must learn quickly
that you cannot turn your sleep on and off like an elec-
tric light switch. Once you have been able to determine
your own sleep needs, you should prepare each day to
approach bedtime so as to adequately allow for the
falling-asleep process. Science has established certain
average patterns for sleep and recognizes the fact that
the older you are the less your sleep needs can be. However, there are other balancing factors. Certainly a man
who works physically all day will require more rest than
one who works mentally. Standard sleep requirements
have been charted for the adult years, and these range
from about eight and one-half hours a day at the
twenty-year-old level to about seven hours a day at the
seventy-year-old level. But these figures may or may not
fit your own cycle best. It is far simpler for you to determine for yourself what your most effective sleep pattern
is. Some people do better to take all their sleep at one
time; others find themselves far more refreshed, and
capable of greater productivity, if they take several cat-

naps during each twenty-four-hour period. And don't think that you can't have too much sleep. Researchers have discovered that some people who have trouble falling asleep do so simply because they are trying to go to bed too early. So the important thing to determine first about your own sleep habits is exactly how much sleep you require. As you have already learned, some people require eight hours, others need only six. Some get by with five or four hours sleep every day. Some people find that a couple of hours sleep two or three times a day is by far the best for their own system.

Of course, married people who find that they have conflicting sleep patterns are likely to encounter serious problems. A man who bounces out of bed at seven in the morning ready to start his day may find that he is ready to fall asleep by eleven in the evening. If his wife has a sleep pattern that keeps her in bed until ten in the morning and then prevents her from falling asleep until one the next morning, there is every reason to believe that this basic difference in sleep pattern can be responsible for many marital conflicts.

What can you do, however, to better your sleep pattern and thus help yourself tune down the emotional stresses of the day? Poor sleep habits, unfortunately, are not cured overnight. The average person who is tense wants to keep on being active. For this reason, people who live under constant stress tend to keep busy far into the night—especially with their mental work.

98

Finally, they hurry to bed and expect to fall asleep immediately. They try, as was pointed out before, to turn sleep off and on. If they cannot—and it is extremely difficult to do—they begin to worry. So their stress and tension is added to with the third destroyer of relaxation: *worry!*

Don't scare
sleep away

Instead of scaring sleep away, you have to try to invite sleep. Perhaps the most conducive invitation to sleep takes place at the bedroom door. At this spot, you should stop and leave your troubles outside. In fact, you ought to begin preparing to drop your troubles at the bedroom door sometime before you even start off into the bedroom. Abstain from talking politics after nine P.M.; do not look at your bankbooks late at night; don't get into arguments in the evening; compose anger and tantrums before you retire. Sleep should, in its own way, be a form of escape. You may even, through sleep, escape for a while from your own company—and that escape will prove to be a lifesaver for you.

If you can allow your mental effort to gradually diminish during the evening, you have established for yourself a psychologically sound approach to the re-

99

laxation that comes in sleep. You should be working at top pressure in the morning. Under the most ideal of circumstances, you should only be working at partial pressure in the afternoon. But certainly, if your afternoon has proved to be more hectic than you anticipated, your evening should be one of low pressure. In this way, you can prepare for the total elimination of pressure which comes in the form of sound sleep. There are odd occasions, undoubtedly, when you must do some serious business in the evening. On those occasions, try to find something to fill in between the business session and the hour that you have set for yourself for sleep. It may be only an easy walk before going to bed. It may be a little time spent at your particular hobby. It may be turning on the record player for some of your favorite music. Whatever it is, you need this to help—as nothing else can—to compensate for the upsetting of your natural-energy rhythm.

Six rules for
a sleep pattern

For the average day, however, there are six basic rules that should help you in establishing an adequate sleep pattern.

The first of these is an attempt to *retire early*. Just as you would with any machine that has been running all day, you must shut off the power. This will allow your fast-moving brain to slowly simmer down to a more relaxed pace. It's the same as a plane coming in for a landing at the airport. The plane cannot discharge its passengers unless it comes down into the airport and to a full stop. You have to do the same thing—come down from the high-flying tension of your day so that you can simmer down into sleep.

Second, as mentioned in the previous chapter, is *exercise*. Your exercise, however, must be well chosen. Vigorous calisthenics are fine for waking up in the morning. They stimulate you. Therefore, they are bad for the pre-sleep period. Similarly, if you take the walk that was suggested earlier, it should not be a brisk walk—unless you can take it long enough before sleep time so that you can allow your muscles to relax. The best exercise before sleep is stretching, followed by yawning and a completely deliberate relaxation of all the muscle groups once you have gotten into bed.

Third is *bathe before bedtime*. However, your baths must be relaxing, not stimulating, ones. A cold bath is a stimulant. And an overly long hot bath will also be a stimulant, because it will stir up your metabolism the same way that a cold bath will. The best way to relax is in a tepid bath, one in which the water temperature is no greater than that of your body—about 100°F. When you get out, pat yourself dry—do not rub vigorously.

Fourth is a rule that many people find difficult to understand and yet one whose true value they appreciate once they try it. This is *a short daytime nap*, or short period in which you lie down to relax. Relaxing once during the day is very conducive to total relaxation—and sleep—once you crawl into bed for the night.

The fifth, a very important rule, is that you should *do nothing stimulating before sleep*. As you have already discovered, arguments are far from being sleep-conducive. Avoid them just as you would avoid a session of listening to rock-and-roll records before sleep time.

The final rule is one that some authors may not like, but it is a good sleep inducer under the right circumstances. It is *reading in bed*—preferably something a little on the dull side. If you read something stimulating, you will only awaken and want to know what is yet to come. You must find something that will take your mind off your other thoughts of the day and yet not stimulate you, so that you can slowly drift into sleep. However this is not going to work if, after you have made yourself drowsy with reading, you then have to get up to brush your teeth and open a window. You must be ready to turn off the light and slide under the covers when you feel that sleep is about to overtake you.

Preparing yourself
for sleep at night

Remember that lying in bed in the quiet darkness with your eyes closed gives you just about the ideal condition for perfect mental concentration. Therefore you must understand the folly of allowing any problem to slip in over the threshold of your mind at that time. If a problem does slip past your defenses, and you have trouble in getting rid of it, open your eyes a little—but keep them relaxed. If your mind is far away, perhaps concentrating on office problems or thinking about what the children did during the day, bring your thoughts back to the problem of sleep and keep it there. Try concentrating on the tip of your own nose. In fact, try looking at your nose—this is an ideal relaxed position for the eyes and eyelids. If you cannot see your nose, perhaps you ought to try introducing subdued light into the room for a time. Perhaps a radio-alarm clock that automatically turns off is a good solution. Turn the radio on to soft music and have your subdued bedside lamp attached to the radio. When the radio turns off automatically, so will the light. Music can be very helpful in avoiding concentration on problems of the day.

If the stressful activity of your day has come to a definite stop, you can be prepared for a restful sleep.

But if your day's stresses have set up self-maintaining tensions, you will be kept awake. If you suffer from insomnia, there is no point in telling yourself, "Forget everything and relax; sleep will come by itself." It will not. Counting sheep, reciting the names of the Presidents of the United States in alphabetical order, and all the other tricks of that type are only of help to those who have faith in them. It is during the whole day that you must prepare yourself for sleep. The day-long preparation involves the following formula which Dr. Selye advocates:

1. Do not allow yourself to get carried away and keyed up more than is necessary to achieve the momentum required in the interest of self-expression. If you get too keyed up, your stress reaction will get carried over into the night and make sleep impossible.

2. Keep in mind that the hormones which produce acute stress are meant to alarm you and key you up for peak accomplishments. They tend to combat sleep and promote alertness during short periods of exertion. They are not meant to be used throughout the day. If too many of these hormones are circulating in your blood, they will keep you awake. Insomnia has a chemical basis which cannot be easily talked away after it has developed. Once you are in bed at night it is too late to prevent it from developing.

3. Realize that variety is the spice of nature. Keep

this in mind not only in planning your day but also in planning your life.

4. Remember, finally, that insomnia is a powerful stressor in itself.

Protect yourself against stress at night, not only by cutting out excesses in light, noise, cold and heat, but by avoiding emotional upsets wherever possible. Avoid getting into a situation of self-perpetuating stress during the day that might automatically continue through the night.

If you can avoid the problem of sleeplessness, you will quickly overcome the companion problem of worry about your inability to sleep. And once you can help yourself overcome worry, you will be well on the way to defeating stress—because worries create stresses.

IV

Stress and Your Heart

8

Worry and Stress

Worry has often been described as the curse of our age. Every one of you is subject to worry, simply because modern life exerts a relentless pressure on all people. There is not one of you who does not feel at times quite inadequate for the burdens and the perplexities of the world. Many people would like to escape from life's responsibilities—but this is not possible, nor is it even desirable. However, the way in which you can carry the responsibilities that life places upon your shoulders does make a vast difference between depression and inadequacy on the one hand and competence and elation on the other.

What is worry? Perhaps it might best be defined as an emotional disturbance which cannot, or which will not, express itself in action. Worry begins as a pinpoint in your emotions—a pinpoint of frustration, a pinpoint of disappointment, a pinpoint of fear, a pinpoint of almost anything in life that develops from a negative reaction to your own progress in any aspect. That pinpoint soon grows, and it grows in every direction. It moves upward, downward, back and forth, sideways, and quickly sets up a jangle that has all our nerves tense and on edge. Before you know it there is an almost continual harshness in your disposition—a harshness that indicates purely and simply that your emotional forces are being used in the wrong way, that they are dashing themselves against obstacles instead of sweeping around those obstacles and cutting out new channels for their own easy flow.

The foundation
of destruction

Doctors and psychiatrists have come to the conclusion that perhaps most of the suffering that people encounter today is due to their worries and, based on worries, all of their fears and their feelings of panic. Most people who worry will readily admit that when they have nothing really to worry about, they make something up simply because they feel happier when they are worrying. Such people are highly illogical. They are the typical "worry-warts" that we all laugh about. Yet how often have you found yourself in a position where you could logically be called a "worry-wart"?

This is not to say that there are not legitimate reasons at times for worry. Nor is it to say that worry can not help to solve some problems. But legitimate or not, worry is the broad foundation of destruction simply because in the long run worry sets up the nervous system to the jangled point of tension at which another "straw" creates damaging stresses.

Worry is a health hazard because it affects three of the body's vital systems: the circulatory, the glandular and the nervous. Each of these systems, in its own way, can play havoc with the heart. You have seen how closely the heart and the circulatory system are connected. You have seen the relationship between the nervous system and the heart. And recent research showed that tension can force the glandular system to bring on heart attacks. This research showed a significant difference in hormone patterns between people who are intensely competitive and those who are more placid. This particular study showed statistically that the highly competitive individuals had seven times as

much coronary artery disease as did their calmer counterparts. The key seems to be in the glandular system—
significant proof from other quarters that Dr. Selye's
theories are sound.

You have probably read in recent years strong denials
that there was any specific basis for the impression that
mental stress or emotional disturbances lay the foundation to coronary artery disease. But simultaneously
various authorities have independently described a
whole series of personality factors in various of their
patients who had heart disease, factors usually sum-
marized in such phrases as "compulsive striving," "hard
work," "self-discipline," and "great need to get to the
top." Of course the tenseness which is so prevalent in
American society today is due to the competitive way
in which we live. And, of course, the "national tension"
has been necessary to create the America that we know
and for which we are grateful. It is clear then, as has
been pointed out to you before, that tension is essential
to living.

Tension keeps you on guard when your safety, well-
being, or self-esteem are threatened. In this respect
it is normal and can be expected from time to time.
However, when emotional upsets—and resulting tension—occur too often, persist, or interfere with everyday living, that is the signal to be on your guard. Most
of these troublesome reactions only concern minor
problems and small disappointments. It is surprising

how often you worry about something that never happens.

Linking stress

to heart ailments

With all this as background, it seems logical that more and more frequently emotional and physical stress should be linked to heart attack. A prime cause of heart and artery attack in reports published in current medical journals is most often stress. A recent ten-year study showed almost conclusively that emotional and physical stress were more often the causes of heart ailments than were heredity and high-fat diets. In pursuing his researches for more than a generation, Dr. Selye has indicated quite clearly that stress is the true origin of degenerative diseases. And included in that list of degenerative diseases are those of the heart and and blood vessels. Through laboratory experiments, Dr. Selye has been able to demonstrate that stress plays a vital role in the development of the heart damage which is known to medical men as cardiac infarcts— the heart "accidents" which account for perhaps half of all the deaths due to heart disease annually. And with this knowledge, Dr. Selye has attempted to find new ways that may lead to prevention of these difficulties, and he has succeeded in many instances. In fact, in his technical book, *The Chemical Prevention of Cardiac Necroses*,[1] he has even indicated a possible cure for these problems.

In the large and busy laboratory at the University of Montreal's School of Medicine, where Dr. Selye and his many assistants labor in their search for the multitudinous effects of stress, there is a vast colony of white rats who daily are exposed to all manner of physical stresses. They are worn down physically by being forced to run in electrically controlled treadmills. They are placed into conditions of intense cold, quickly followed by intense heat. They are tossed about in chicken-wire rollers and then immobilized on boards. Everything is done to build up their stress to the point where their glandular system is affected. The result has been that the hormone mechanisms have reached the point where the animals have had created in them an acute, spontaneous lesion in the heart muscle—a lesion almost identical to a heart infarct in a human.

Dr. Selye has been able to develop large and clearly visible yellowish patches of dead tissue on the vital heart muscle simply by having certain chemicals injected into the rat and then exposing the animal to sudden and extreme stress. It is obvious then, since rats are very much like humans, with the same adrenal

[1] *The Chemical Prevention of Cardiac Necroses*, Hans Selye, The Ronald Press Company, New York, 1958.

and pituitary glands, that the stress-produced heart damage in the animal is virtually identical to heart damage produced by stress in humans.

The chemical basis

for heart damage

Will these experiments be useful to mankind? Does what happens to rats happen to men? Dr. Selye hopes so simply because his experiments have not only been worked successfully on rats and cats, dogs and hamsters, but also monkeys—the closest laboratory animal to man. It is Dr. Selye's feeling that, of all his work, this discovery might possibly be the most immediately practical and the most likely to help ailing humans. To boil down several hundred pages of chemical formulas and highly technical medical language, Dr. Selye's theory is that a man who is weakened by an imbalance of hormones and various chemicals—that is, "salts"—in his body and who is then subjected to additional outside stresses may develop a sudden heart attack and die quite unexpectedly from the cardiac infarct. What this means is that the supply of blood to part of the heart muscle has been blocked. The muscle, therefore, is not being fed with the oxygen it requires to continue its job of pumping blood to the rest of the body. Thus starved, it dies. While such infarcts, or accidents, sometimes follow blocking of a coronary artery, this is not the only cause of a cardiac infarct. Such an accident can occur, Dr. Selye points out, when the heart has become starved for blood by some unusual physical exertion or other outside tension creating a vast amount of stress and demanding abnormal amounts of blood for some other part of the body.

Dr. Selye notes that a common belief is that sudden exertion will bring on a heart attack which is fatal. In the area of Canada where his laboratory is, heavy snowstorms are not infrequent during the winter months. Many a man forced to shovel snow, and unaccustomed to such hard labor, collapses and dies later in the day. Such deaths are usually attributed to a heart attack. Dr. Selye says, however, that the victim has been killed by stress. And stress is the guilty party in countless other deaths of people who are not accustomed to strenuous physical activity and who are forced into such situations.

Of course, with good medical care, with rest and with the proper medication, perhaps four-fifths of all people survive such an attack the first time. However, of those who survive about fifteen per cent will suffer the second attack within one year and more than fifty per cent of those who have had a heart infarct are likely to die within three to five years from subsequent "accidents" of this sort.

The significance of Dr. Selye's work, however, is double-barreled. While, in the first place, he has discovered that powerful chemicals—a hormone (methylchlorocortisol) and phosphates—lay the foundation to a weakened heart that can be destroyed by stress, he has concomitantly discovered that injections of other chemicals can protect against stress. In his further experiments, Dr. Selye gave his animals magnesium and potassium salts which counteracted the death-dealing chemicals and reduced the incidence of death from this form of cardiac necrosis. Dr. Selye hopes that, since both of these chemicals are safe and well-known, a practical and effective mixture can be developed that can be administered under your physician's supervision so that your body can distribute them slowly and gradually and help combat the dangers of stress.

Anxieties cause tensions and if you cannot express your tension in words or deeds then, much like steam under pressure, these tensions will express themselves as symptoms. Important as anxiety is in relation to the heart that is normal, it is even more important to people suffering from heart disease. Anxiety can impose a physiological burden on the overworked heart, a burden that is too much for even the strongest heart to live with.

Stresses, anxieties, and tensions—all can play havoc with the heart and the circulatory system. Emotional stress cannot be measured. It has no meaning except in relation to you under your own particular stress. Nor does emotional stress, tension, or anxiety depend upon external circumstances in which you find yourself; they all depend upon your ability to handle such stressful situations. If worries plague and get the better of you, the resulting fears and anxieties instantly mobilize the body's defense mechanisms. This defensive reaction involves a sudden flooding of the blood with the hormone adrenalin. Adrenalin shortens the clotting time of blood and so can lead to the easier formation of clots in the coronary artery. Stress may increase the cholesterol content of the blood. It may also produce an increase in the fatty deposit in the coronary arteries. Fear can produce significant changes in an electrocardiogram. Steady pressure of nerve impulses can affect the tone of the coronary artery. It is obvious, therefore, that regardless of what mechanism is affected, emotional factors can, and will, increase the chances for a heart attack.

On this foundation of emotional stress need only be laid the "last straw" of physical stress and the body's vital organ is ready to be made an easy victim—a victim of worry!

9

Stress and Coronary Thrombosis

The chances are that even before you opened the first page of this book you understood the terms "heart attack" and "heart disease." They are terms that are most often used to indicate a physiological process in which, by one means or another, one of the coronary arteries has been closed off. Actually, there are four different medical terms that can be used to describe a "heart attack," and they don't all mean the same thing.

The one term that is probably most familiar to you is "coronary thrombosis." Often, however, "coronary closure" and "coronary occlusion" will be used more or less synonymously for coronary thrombosis. Another frequently used term is "myocardial infarction." This is not quite synonymous with the others inasmuch as a myocardial infarction may occur without coronary thrombosis, and the other way around as well. Of the four terms, perhaps the last one needs some further explanation, since it is strictly medical terminology. Myocardium is a Latin word which means heart muscle; it is the word which most doctors prefer when talking of that muscle. The word infarction, as you have already learned in an earlier chapter, means that tissue has suddenly died as a result of complete loss of its blood supply.

Why should the blood supply be cut off suddenly? There are a number of reasons, among them a "thrombus," or blood clot; an "embolus," or matter that is foreign to the blood stream but not necessarily a blood clot; and an "atheroma," or granules of fattiness. If any one of these prevents blood from being supplied to one or more areas of the body, the tissue will not survive for very long. When the blood supply is cut off by a stoppage in the arterial system and the heart muscle does not get its life-giving blood, those muscle fibers will die and be replaced by scar tissue.

Younger people
are being affected

Coronary thrombosis is not merely a matter of arteries that are becoming older and whose walls are becoming thicker, thus narrowing the vital channels through which blood must pass. In fact, with greater and greater frequency, coronary thrombosis is happening to younger people. And surveys indicate that heart attacks are found more frequently among men who are always harried, hurried, and overworked and who are plagued by many business problems, or among ambitious people who drive themselves hard and allow their obligations to interfere with normal rest. The man who is unhappy and restless at home is a common victim. So is the constant worrier, the man who has permitted everyday stresses to wear down his system into premature aging.

But even with the increasing stresses of modern life, it is still unfair to say that there has been a noticeable increase in coronary thrombosis. It is unfair simply because a complete study could never be undertaken. Many people have heart attacks—mild ones—that go unrecognized and can never be counted. It is, nevertheless, still safe to say that the rapid pace of modern life has put abnormal strain on the heart and in consequence more people suffer from heart disease. You must also consider the fact that if coronary thrombosis is more common than it used to be it is because you are living longer than your forefathers did. This is a disease that, although it strikes younger men, does occur more frequently in those who are older.

Men are affected by this disease four times as frequently as women. And, while older people are the ones who are the most susceptible to coronary thrombosis, in the thirties and forties five men are stricken to every two women. In the late forties, the chances are four to one that a man will be stricken with coronary thrombosis than a woman. And even in the sixties and seventies, twice as many men die of this form of heart attack as do women. It seems to go almost without saying that the price of success in the present-day world is coronary heart disease.

In looking for the causes of coronary thrombosis and all the related diseases, medical men have more and more begun to point the accusing finger at three factors: heredity, high-fat diets and emotional strain. And more and more the dangers of stress have been emphasized in the results of many reseachers' work into the kinds of personalities which are most prone to heart attack. One leading consultant in heart research has gone so far as to say that even the "lethalness of a high-fat diet in our society seems to be dependent on the 'catalytic influence' of stressful living."

The stress-blind
personality type

The difficulty is that there are people whom we might call "stress blind." They are people who do not recognize the limit to which their own bodies can react successfully to stress. People of this sort are usually compulsive about time. They are overworked. They burn with desire to be recognized. They are the people who are constantly restless during their leisure hours and usually feel very guilty about not working at those times.

The stress-blind personality is a perfectionist. He is extremely impatient with those who work under him. He is very over-meticulous and prefers to do work himself rather than to delegate it to others. The interesting factor is that it is not his job alone that produces the stress in him. More frequently, the stress comes from multiple goals that he has set for himself and this is combined with his own attitudes toward these goals. As in all areas of life, people seek to compensate for anxieties. The stress-blind personality compensates in an unfortunate manner. He overeats, he smokes to excess, he drinks far too much, and above all he commits himself so heavily to business and social obligations that he has no time for exercise. What happens? The answer is quite simple and understandable. He sets up within himself a mechanism by which his glands provide the body with extra fuel for his extraordinary effort. Because these stress-blind people are constantly striving and are constantly frustrated, their bodies react as though they were constantly carrying a burden. The result is that there is a great increase in blood cholesterol and in fatty molecules in the blood stream. These in turn increase the danger of thrombosis particularly when the other factors—such as heredity and a high-fat diet—are already present.

The United States Air Force, in recent research, discovered that in certain instances of emotional stress, the cholesterol level in some people was actually doubled. These emotional stresses were not always the kinds of anxieties that could be described as acute rage. They were more often normal stresses—stresses that are encountered in taking over a new job, or in working to get projects ready to meet deadlines, or in situations such as a man might encounter in preparing a report for the approval of two groups with opposing views. Nor was it found in these studies that men at the executive level had higher cholesterol content in their systems than others. All in all, however, in the group that the Air Force study covered, coronary disease was found to be more prevalent in those men with the highest cholesterol content in their system. It appeared that the cholesterol build-up in the blood could act very much in the same way as an oily rag left in an unused corner of the closet. It will burn if the proper source of ignition becomes present—a kind of spontaneous combustion.

Stress boosts
cholesterol content

Studies by the American Medical Association have established statistically that elevated blood levels of cholesterol, the fatty substance which is present as a normal and essential part of the human body, are found to be associated with heart disease. In fact, it is believed that high cholesterol content is responsible for more than ninety-five per cent of all coronary heart disease. Whether fatty foods are harmful, however, is a matter of great controversy. Whether the fatty factor in blood runs in families is also a controversial point in medical research. But these factors are not of prime importance at this juncture—the important factor about cholesterol content is twofold. First, it is well established that it is the trigger for the great majority of heart disease. Second, it is well established that stress can boost the cholesterol level in your body to abnormal proportions.

The Air Force studies clearly indicated that cholesterol and fat concentrations in the blood increase under stress—and return to normal values after the stressful periods are over. As a result of these studies, it became obvious that people have to be educated to take regular exercise and to reduce the fat content in their diet. It was obvious, too, that people have to be taught the effects of stress and the need for eliminating stressful reactions in their daily lives. Another study made some years ago on the West Coast had even more startling results in determining how quickly blood will clot under stressful conditions. A group of accountants, all men, were checked over a six-month period during which time the income tax deadline approached and passed. It was found that blood cholesterol levels were highest during the pre-deadline rush for more than eighty per cent of the group. When these men were under the least stress, their blood-clotting time averaged a little under ten minutes. When the work was hardest, however, the blood clotted in about half that time. Obviously, the faster that your blood coagulates, the more quickly it can form a clot. And the more readily that clots form, the more likely becomes the possibility of coronary thrombosis.

Overwork, as such, is not necessarily the major factor in stress as it affects the statistics of coronary thrombosis. The stresses of the job may only be part of the problem. There can be stresses at home—arguments with a wife, arguments between a wife and children, criticism by a husband, unhappy social situations and obligations. At almost all times, stress of emotional origin accompanies stress of overwork. And the stress of overwork, in itself, is likely to be a killer. The two stresses together are like an automobile running with the emergency brake on. The emotional stress is the emergency brake, and this must be released. But the automobile must keep running. The body requires exercise—not excessive tranquility. Comparative studies made between active workers and sedentary workers have indicated time after time that coronary thrombosis is found less frequently among those persons who are active. It is the emotional stress, then, that increases the work of the heart. You have only to note your own increased heart rate during excitement to know that this statement is true.

Under emotional stress influences, physiological changes may be brought about that increase the work of the heart and impair its efficiency. Emotional factors undoubtedly add to the burden that your heart is conditioned to carry—but too often they add more than it is able to support.

10

Anxiety and Angina Pectoris

Angina pectoris, the stabbing heart pain, is definitely known to be a warning that blood supply to the heart is not sufficient for its needs. The pain of angina, severe though it may be at times, can actually serve as a life-saver. For this pain warns the victim that the time has come to let up in his activities and especially that he should avoid acute emotional upsets which put severe stress upon the heart.

Angina pectoris is called by many names. You may hear it referred to simply as angina, or perhaps anginal heart failure. It may be called cardiac pain, or coronary pain, or simply heart pain. In a sense, the word angina is misleading since it comes from the word *angere*, which is Latin for strangle. And the pain that accompanies an attack of angina has also been described in misleading ways. You may have heard people describe an anginal pain as being unbearable and paralyzing. Medical research, however, indicates that these descriptions are inaccurate and usually untrue. If the symptoms are severe, unbearable pain, accompanied by difficulty in breathing and profuse sweating, the chances are that the victim has suffered a heart attack—a thrombosis— and not angina.

Doctors are agreed that the pain from angina is, in most cases, a pressure or a squeezing—a kind of tightness rather than any actual pain. It is as though you buckled your belt too tight and found that your breathing became difficult. The onset of this aching and burning feeling is seldom sudden. The pain seems to build up gradually and get worse. While the entire attack may last only a few minutes—rarely more than five minutes—it seems to the sufferer that the pain has been there for a very long time.

It is interesting to note, from the point of view of the effect that anxiety can have on angina, that if the sufferer should stop all his activity at the first indication that a seizure is coming on there will be no pain developing. It is true that there will be some slight soreness in the chest that may last for perhaps thirty or forty minutes. But it is equally true that, unlike other kinds of pain, the attack of angina ceases promptly when the victim rests and remains absolutely quiet and free of emotional anxiety.

The warning
goes unheeded

Angina is actually the result of an inadequate flow of blood through the coronary arteries. It is, in effect, an advance warning of more serious heart disease. Unfortunately, it is a warning that frequently goes unheeded. Too often, tragically, victims have not recognized the pains for the warning attacks that they are and have therefore not consulted a doctor before a major coronary attack has begun its deadly work.

What is the warning? Simply that in the case of angina the heart muscle is deprived of blood for a very short time—at most, perhaps, only five minutes. It is a warning, therefore, that this deprivation can occur again in more serious form. When the heart muscle is deprived of blood for a long period of time—or permanently—then coronary thrombosis is the result.

It is obvious that angina is brought about when fatty deposits—deposits of cholesterol—build up in the coronary artery, or in smaller arterial passages that lead to the heart, and temporarily cause a cessation of life-giving blood flow to the body pump.

When this happens, discomfort quickly occurs in the center of the chest, in the front, somewhere behind the breastbone, and sometimes fairly low or fairly high. While the pain itself seems to be directly over the heart, in virtually all cases the heart has nothing to do with the resulting pain of an angina attack. Often the pain moves into the throat with a sense of choking. Sometimes it moves to a shoulder and down the arm as far as the elbow, or even further. And while it may move into either arm, it more frequently is felt in the left shoulder and arm. The pain may even be felt in the side of the face and along the jaw.

The frequency of anginal attacks will vary greatly from one person to another. Most patients claim to have only occasional attacks that are weeks or sometimes even months apart. Others, however, experience them quite regularly and even sometimes as often as once a day. But, as has been pointed out, if the patient learns to relax and especially to avoid particular kinds of exertion, the attacks can be avoided with almost as much regularity as they might occur.

It is important to note that a twinge in the vicinity of your heart does not necessarily mean that there has been an angina attack. There are many conditions that cause chest pain and can be mistaken for angina. Anxiety, while one of the chief causes of angina, is also a possible cause, in itself, of sharp and sticking pains that are frequently felt around the heart. Oddly enough, the pain from anxiety, coupled with fatigue and nervous tension, may even spread in much the same fashion that the anginal pain will. However, the pain brought on by anxiety is usually felt on the side of the chest where the tip of the heart lies and is never felt under the breast-bone as is an actual angina seizure. Pain from anxiety occurs usually after exertion or even after excitement. The pain from angina will strike *during* exertion or excitement.

The important thing to remember, however, is that you should not be the one to decide what a pain in your chest means or what it has been caused by. This is a decision that should—and must—be left to your doctor.

When angina
may strike

When does angina strike? Usually in the middle years or beyond. Perhaps more than ninety per cent of sufferers of anginal pain have already lived more than forty years, and some three-fourths of them are beyond the age of fifty. Again, angina strikes at men more frequently than it does at women. Various studies place

132

the ratio at anywhere between three angina attacks for men to one for women, and as many as six to one.

As in the case of other diseases of the heart, individuals who are likely to suffer an anginal attack are those whose workloads are fertile grounds for anxiety. Angina patients are often aggressive people, over-ambitious ones, individuals who tend toward emotional excesses. They are people who are quick-tempered more often than not.

Next to physical exercise as the prime cause of bringing on an attack of angina, anxiety ranks a strong second. Of course, you have discovered by now that emotional tension is the equivalent of exercise as far as the heart is concerned. Anxieties, tensions, worries, all of these cause the heart to beat faster and the blood pressure to rise. This faster beating—sometimes incredibly faster—coupled with the increase in pressure in the arterial system increases the workload of the heart. Surprisingly, these effects may take place within a matter of seconds, and they highlight how anxiety pressures the system into the first step on the road to physical breakdown.

When anxiety is the direct cause of an attack of angina, the duration of the pain is likely to be far greater. Anxieties brought on by anger, by misfortune, by distress, these create an internal storm that cannot be quelled in a matter of a few minutes. Since the factor that causes the anxiety is a continuing one, the pain itself is likely to continue for periods that may last as long as a quarter of an hour.

As greater and greater requirements are demanded of you in almost every field of activity, you find that you are denied the necessary long hours of quiet contemplation, recreation—and even insulation from your surroundings—which are conducive to combating failure of the blood-pumping system. Each time your body is subjected to the pressures of emotional stress that demand physical response, extra blood is required. To get this extra blood through the body, your heart will pump at emergency speed—but if your arteries are not healthy, if they have been clogging up with fatty "rusts," then angina is likely. If your coronary arteries, distorted and narrowed by accumulations of fat, are unable to deliver the added nourishment and the supply of fresh oxygen that is essential for each emergency, the heart strains and struggles. So the emotional stress can cause physical strain—and the victim consciously knows quite suddenly that something has gone wrong. Pain tells him.

The heart stricken by angina is no different than the retired taxicab with more than 100,000 miles on it. If you don't race that car, or slam-bang it over rough roads, or try to drive it like a "hot rod," there are countless miles still available from it. It can be used steadily —but it has to be used reasonably.

Your heart, attacked by stress, is no different.

134

11

Tension and Sclerosis

Sclerosis—because of the morbid effects it can have upon the heart—is by far the leading cause of death not only in the United States but probably in most other countries of Western civilization.

The word sclerosis is not really a common one—though most of you have undoubtedly read at least some literature on arteriosclerosis. The word sclerosis comes from a Greek word which means hard. And, in effect, any of the sclerotic conditions do mean a hardening. However, it might be easier to conceive of coronary sclerosis as a scarring of the arteries and consequently a loss of their ability to nourish the heart properly. It is, as was pointed out previously, as though scaly rust gathers in the arterial pipes and begins to clog them with coat after coat of waste material that is built up with each new deposit. The arterial pipes—in the same manner as water pipes—become narrower and narrower on the inside and eventually only a trickle of blood can get through. When the heart cannot get blood except in a trickle, the heart tissue is bound to suffer—as you have already seen. So arteriosclerosis, and the various other forms of sclerotic arteries, will lead to coronary thrombosis and ultimately to death.

Cholesterol
and sclerosis

Because the key, therefore, to the fatal attack—thrombosis—lies with sclerosis, the reason for this sclerotic condition of the arteries is perhaps the most important medical question confronting science today. And while medical researchers are inclined to agree that perhaps no single factor will explain adequately all the known facts relating to this serious disease, there is no doubt that among the five principal reasons which might predispose you to arteriosclerosis—and eventual heart attack—is an elevated blood cholesterol level.

136

It would be unfair to discuss one cause for arteriosclerosis and dismiss the others. Therefore, before going on to the problem of cholesterol and sclerosis, the other four key reasons should be discussed in brief.

Heredity is the first of these. It has been found that coronary heart disease is nearly four times as prevalent among brothers and sisters of people who have had coronary artery disease as among brothers and sisters of people who have not had it. Dr. M. M. Gertler and his associates, in a study made some years ago, said, "It is reasonable to suspect the existence of hereditary genetic factors in the etiology of coronary heart disease." This report added that it was reasonable to conclude that coronary heart disease was more likely to occur in families or individuals if the mother, the father, or brothers and sisters had experienced the disease previously.

The second possible reason is *obesity*—or more simply, overweight. Studies in recent years have shown a significant difference in the amount of coronary disease among people who are overweight as compared to people who are underweight. The harmful influence of obesity on the normal—as well as on the diseased— heart has been well established by many medical researchers. Dr. Leonid Kotkin, in his book *Eat, Think and Be Slender*[1] says, "Arteriosclerosis, high blood pres-

[1] *Eat, Think and Be Slender,* Leonid Kotkin, Hawthorn Books, New York, 1954.

sure . . . heart disease . . . are more prevalent and more serious in overweight individuals." It has been estimated that the risk of myocardial infarction—the "accident" that occurs when the blood supply is cut off from the heart tissue—is increased by about fifty per cent due to overweight and about seventy per cent due to hypertension.

The third reason is *increased blood pressure*. The sclerotic complications are two to three times more common in persons whose blood pressure has been elevated unduly. One study recently published showed that in men between the ages of forty-five and sixty-two, elevation of blood pressure was associated very definitely with the development of coronary heart disease.

Fourthly, there is the contributing factor of *excessive smoking*. Any number of studies have proved that a susceptibility to sclerotic conditions can be linked to excessive use of tobacco. A series of studies done over a period of years with the same people showed that men with a history of regular cigarette smoking have a considerably higher death rate than those who have never smoked, and disease of the coronary arteries was indicated as the primary cause of death.

These four factors, along with an increased cholesterol level in the blood, are believed on the basis of scientific evidence to be the principal causes of sclerosis. Since it has already been shown conclusively that the cholesterol level can be increased considerably by tension, it is obvious that stresses on the body definitely damage the coronary arteries. One study of several hundred men with established myocardial infarction showed that their cholesterol level was much higher, on the average, than that of a similar group of men of similar age without obvious disease. Cholesterol has definitely been shown to be present at a much higher frequency and at much higher concentrations in patients who have survived a myocardial infarction than in corresponding people in whom no known heart disease, or arterial disease, exists. A British study found that "The concentration of cholesterol . . . is increased in a group of men with coronary sclerosis when contrasted with a group of normal men of comparable age."

The commonest form of sclerosis

The most common, and the most serious, form of arteriosclerosis has already been mentioned—that is, atherosclerosis. Your doctor may refer to it as "atheromatosis." This word is often used because the basic change in the artery consists of the formation of what are called "atheromas" in its inner lining, or "intima." The word atheroma comes from a Greek word which means groats or porridge. It is used because the condition is a kind of tumorous one that resembles porridge in a way. It is really a deposit on the inner lining of the artery which contains fatty substances that include cholesterol. The atheromas usually do not remain small. In fact, they increase in size rather rapidly because of connective tissue that grows between them, and this results in the change which is known as sclerosis. Often there is a chemical deposit—usually lime salts—and this is known as calcification. These deposits, as they become larger, cause the decrease in the size of the channel through which the blood flows. In addition, the surface of the inner lining of the artery is no longer smooth and the irregular rough spots provide more favorable conditions for clotting of the blood upon it.

When the circulation has been finally reduced by atherosclerosis to such an extent that the condition can be easily recognized, then you will find that doctors may use any number of names to describe it. These sclerotic conditions might be called coronary atherosclerosis or coronary artery disease. They may be labeled coronary heart disease, atherosclerotic heart disease, or arteriosclerotic heart disease. The name by which your doctor calls it, however, is not important. The fact of vital importance is that in the average male older than twenty-five there is very likely to be a condition of atherosclerosis present. In other words, this condition does exist under normal circumstances. The main point to be remembered, then, is that this condition can be heightened and made more dangerous by tension, by anxiety, by stress, by worry, by anything that will increase the output of cholesterol into the blood stream. It is a scientific fact that the atherosclerosis may appear earlier, and progress far more rapidly, if the patient suffers from hypertension.

Many of you may jump to the conclusion that since fatty deposits are the catalytic agent to sclerosis, the problem would be simple if fat-rich diets were avoided. This is by no means the case, unfortunately. Many people have consumed vast quantities of fat-rich foods and have survived to a ripe old age with no coronary symptoms whatsoever. On the other hand, people with a complete aversion to fatty foods do occasionally develop the disease. Therefore you cannot point the guilty finger solely at a fat-rich diet, despite the fact that fatty substances building up on the arterial walls do the basic damage. The problem is simply that all people are different. And the differences in their coronary arteries are perhaps as wide as the differences in their fingerprints. Some arteries are able to handle fatty substances better than others. The individual differences are further complicated by the fact that at varied times and under varied circumstances people react differently from each other. Again, we come back to the problem of tensions as they affect the entire circulatory system. Each one of you reacts differently to tension. Each one of you suffers from stresses in different intensities, at different times, under different circumstances. A complex of factors adds up to a giant question mark—there is no saying how much tension your body can take without creating irreparable damage to the arterial system.

And while many people have weathered extremely stressful situations without evidence of excessive damage from heart disease, it is quite well established that when a patient who already has a well-developed degree of atherosclerosis involving key arteries of the heart suddenly suffers acute stress—such as is commonly seen shortly after a great personal tragedy, for instance —a severe coronary attack is bound to occur.

The "villain" is atherosclerosis—or arteriosclerosis— caused by the lining and subsequent narrowing of the arteries with cholesterol and calcium and the clotting of the blood which prevents the flow of proper food supply to the heart muscle. The "devil," constantly standing behind the villain and prodding him endlessly, is stress.

12

Hypertension:

High Blood Pressure

There is a great deal of confusion over just what high blood pressure is. Perhaps one of the greatest causes of this confusion is that there is no set "normal pressure." Blood pressure varies with your age, your state of mind, and the presence or absence of other disease. What may be dangerous to one person may have little significance to you. However, what your doctor means by high blood pressure—and what he is looking for when he puts a blood-pressure cuff around your arm in what may be a routine physical examination—is the pressure that is, all things considered, too high and stays too high for *you.* The reason for this is that sustained high pressure is damaging to your blood vessels and to your heart. Sustained high blood pressure hastens hardening of the arteries and compels the heart to work harder. Thus it leads to heart failure and contributes greatly to coronary heart disease. Two out of every fifteen deaths in the United States have been directly attributed to high blood pressure. And while it is no respecter of persons, it is more frequent in women than it is in men—though, since you have already seen that heart disease is more frequent in men, high blood pressure is consequently more lethal in the male.

High blood pressure, or hypertension as it is called, is most common in people during the forties and the early fifties. It does, however, occur in the thirties and may even occur in the twenties. What is the cause of hypertension? The term itself is almost self-explanatory. The prefix "hyper" means intense; therefore, hypertension is intensified tension. It is strain almost to the point of breaking. Faulty diet is certainly one of the possible causes of hypertension, since your blood pressure is affected by overweight. But more important are the psychological factors that play a part in building up the pressure of the blood to the point of causing arterial and heart damage.

It is commonly known that emotional excitement can send the blood pressure shooting skyward. In fact, the

144

responsiveness of blood pressure to emotion makes it difficult for the physician to obtain readings that accurately reflect a patient's true blood pressure. The fact is that when you visit the doctor's office, your emotional reaction to such a visit might be sufficient in itself to send your blood pressure way above normal.

Picture of a
hypertensive person

However, there is a picture into which most hypertensive persons fit: They are high-strung, hard-driving, conscientious people. The hypertensive patient is likely to be irritable and to have sharp emotional ups-and-downs. The difficulty is that he usually bottles up his emotions and keeps a calm front to the rest of the world, at least when he is away from home—in his office, at social gatherings and, worst of all, in the doctor's office.

An important key as to how stresses affect the hypertensive person was found in a study at Johns Hopkins University. This study showed that the heart muscle, just as all other muscles of the body, can "learn" and can even form habits. Therefore, a man whose life has been marked by times of repeated stress, during which his heart obviously had to beat faster and his blood pressure was forced to rise, may find himself suffering

145

from high blood pressure even though the causative stress itself has vanished. The difficulty is that his heart has learned a habit all too well. It keeps on acting as though it were still under the same excitement. So the hypertensive patient is often a difficult one to recognize. He keeps a calm face to the outward world and does not show the boiling that goes on within him. And when his stresses have passed, his heart muscle, having learned its bad habits too well, keeps on reacting in a way that is unfavorable to his general condition.

Unfortunately, hypertension may produce no outward symptoms for years for this simple reason. And even when symptoms do develop, the patient may get along quite well for ten or even twenty years—perhaps longer. But the symptoms that do present themselves—and they can be any of a vast multitude—are usually due to anxiety, to fear, or to nervous tension, even when the blood pressure is normal. Furthermore, the severity of the symptoms that do present themselves need not necessarily parallel the degree of rise in blood pressure.

Moreover, the heart in long-standing severe hypertension works under a double disadvantage. There is a tendency for the coronary arteries to become hard and their channels to become narrowed, as has already been explained. A diminished blood supply results, and the heart muscle gets reduced nourishment and energy so that its pumping action is less efficient. The heart, as

146

you have seen, is a sturdy organ. It often copes adequately with such disadvantages—sometimes even for years—so that no symptoms develop. When symptoms do develop, they may take the form of shortness of breath during simple and ordinary exertion. There may be palpitation, a little cough at night, or even some pain in the region of the heart—especially on walking, or after a heavy meal, or during excitement.

Recent research at the University of Texas has pointed a finger at another possible cause of hypertension and high blood pressure—again a cause that is the result of stress. This research links high blood pressure with poor kidney blood supply. The kidney, just as are all the other of the body's organs, is supplied with blood nourishment to keep it functioning. When the arteries leading to the kidney get choked up, however, then the blood supply is partially shut off in the same manner as the blood supply to the heart can be shut off. The blockage of these arteries is no different than the blockage of the arteries that lead to the heart. Fatty deposits, caused by stresses, build up in these arteries just as they do in all other arteries. The Texas researchers showed that a blood-starved kidney of this kind gets local help when it calls for more blood. However, this local help is usually at the cost of increasing blood pressure throughout the entire body, thus contributing to the causes of heart damage.

147

How high must high blood pressure be to become dangerous? Perhaps not as high as medical science once thought. A recent analysis of deaths over a twenty-year period indicated that relatively small blood-pressure elevations in apparently healthy people carry a far more significant mortality risk than had previously been supposed. This evidence, then, unfortunately points to the fact that there is no place on the blood-pressure scale which can be called the last safe level to which blood pressure can rise. Nor is there a cutoff point at which a person with only mild hypertension is safe from the deadly action that occurs in the arterial system and in the heart.

Your nerves

and hypertension

There are many studies which indicate quite clearly that the nervous system may play an important part in the development of hypertension in some people. One of the earliest changes that can be seen in people suffering from hypertension is a widespread constricting of the arterioles, the smallest branches of the arteries which, as you have learned, have muscular walls that are capable of contracting and thus forcing blood through them. This contraction, however, is controlled by nerve impulses. These impulses come through the autonomic nervous system which also keeps most of the body's vital functions in constant operation. This is the nervous system over which you have no control and which, therefore, maintains your bodily functions during sleep or anesthesia, and controls the automatic activities of the various organs. Research has shown that it is reasonably certain that when fear, anxiety, tension, or stress occurs, the nervous system is affected to the point that the arterioles are constricted—and the end result is an increase in blood pressure in much the same way as you would build up the pressure in a garden hose if you were to squeeze the tubing flat at several points and only allow a trickle of water through.

The early phases of hypertension seem to reflect an abnormal and excessive responsiveness of the blood vessels and nerves to the strain of life. Sometimes—as for instance during military battles—the hypertension is much more severe when the strain is extraordinary. Yet it may pass off after the emergency. But when your nervous system reacts violently to ordinary events, every day becomes a succession of emergencies and your blood pressure progressively becomes higher and tends more and more to remain so. However, even in the later stages of high blood pressure, nervous factors continue to play an important part. Doctors use the simple test of plunging a patient's hand into ice water. In a normal person, the resulting cold and pain cause the blood pressure to rise. But in a hypertensive person, the blood pressure usually rises far more than in the case of a normal person. Since the sensation of pain or cold is carried from the hand to the central nervous system, it is reasonable to suppose that the excessive rise in blood pressure indicates an excitable nervous system. You don't have to be a physician—or even a sufferer of high blood pressure—to be aware of the role that your nervous system plays in blood pressure. You have undoubtedly experienced a pounding of the heart that goes with excitement. You feel that your blood pressure is elevated at such a time—and you are quite right.

When is the danger

point reached?

But the nervous system is not the only part of the body that can increase blood pressure. The glands, too, can be stimulated to secrete substances that appear in the mechanisms of hypertension—and you have already learned how stresses affect the glandular system of the body.

The chief danger of persistent hypertension is arteriosclerosis. The amount of scarring in the walls of the arteries and arterioles depends upon several factors. The first of these is how high the pressure is. Secondly, and a little more important, is the length of time during which the pressure has been elevated. Lastly—and by far the most important factor—is the ability of the blood vessels to stand the strain.

You have already learned how the walls of the arteries become scarred, what the effects are, and how a certain amount of sclerosis develops in nearly everyone as age increases. High blood pressure, however, speeds and intensifies these changes. Sustained hypertension increases the susceptibility of the coronary arteries to sclerosis. The heart soon begins to falter—though the patient will not be noticeably inconvenienced by high blood pressure. The heart muscle grows larger and stronger in an effort to maintain the high blood pressure. At first it is more efficient, but the time comes when the growth of new blood vessels to nourish the enlarging fibers of the heart muscle does not keep pace. So the enlarged heart is deprived of adequate food, just as the heart can be starved when the coronary arteries become obstructed by clots or narrowing. The heart reacts just as would a ditchdigger trying to get along on a filing clerk's diet. Instead of getting a larger supply of blood to nourish its greater bulk, the heart receives less. Its efficiency drops and soon the signs of serious heart disease appear.

It seems likely that the word "tension" is an important part of the term hypertension with some reason. It has been said that medical men, before the discovery of high blood pressure, diagnosed the symptoms as "bad temper." There is no doubt that there is an important relationship of emotional stress to the onset of hypertension and to the anxiety which is frequently responsible for aggravation of existing high blood pressure. Personality studies of high-blood-pressure cases have often revealed deep-seated emotional conflicts which stand in close relationship to this anxiety. And while some people may be born with a marked predisposition to high blood pressure, there is no doubt that stress is a key factor in bringing it to a head. Those who seem predisposed to hypertension probably require only little environmental stress. Others probably require a considerable degree of environmental stress to bring about tension. Whichever type the patient is, it is clear that hypertension begins with temporary elevations of blood pressure in response to stresses during the earlier years and becomes established at higher levels because of continuing stress in the later years. At its final stage it becomes fixed at a level which doctors call "essential hypertension"—the word essential here meaning unknown, or of unknown origin.

V

Your Defense
Against Stress

13

Hostility and Hypertension

There was a mythical king of Corinth called Sisyphus. Sisyphus was forever condemned to roll a boulder up a mountain, only to have it slip from his grasp within a hair's breadth of the summit, so that his travails had to be endlessly repeated. But poor King Sisyphus suffered no greater frustrations in his daily tasks than most of you. Life is full of frustrating experiences—frustrations that go on day after day, month after month, year after year, frustrations that continue despite the fact that you meet many successes along the road.

The average man or woman is constantly troubled with everyday frustrations: the continual striving to get ahead, the continual driving to meet deadlines, the desire for recognition and advancement. These all set up a tempo of living—both in the business world and in the social world—that make for serious difficulty as the body tries to cope with stress. There is no evidence that demanding executive occupations are the only ones that are stressful. Hard work, and all that goes with it, is common to men of all social classes. Chronic stress is part and parcel of the day-to-day program of every-one's life. You see examples all about you of stresses, stresses imposed from the outside and stresses imposed from within the individual himself.

From the outside there are such pressures as those imposed by an employer, a spouse, or by status-seeking with all its pressures and frustrations. From the inside, you have seen people who carry on running battles with clerks, doormen, fellow workers, even their own families. They live with an "Old Man of the Sea" on their shoulders. Not only are they stressful all of their waking hours, sometimes they are stressful even while they are asleep.

Stress is, therefore, a part of everyone's everyday life. As Dr. Selye has tried to underline, stress is not all negative. But, when it is unduly prolonged, or when it comes too often, or when it is concentrated on one particular organ or part of the body—then trouble is bound to appear. The glands will produce too much of one hormone, or not enough of another. The concept of stress has changed the entire understanding of the process of aging. Aging is no longer determined by the time elapsed since birth. It is now determined by the total amount of wear and tear to which your body is exposed. It is as though at birth every one of you inherited a certain amount of physical adaptive energy. You can draw upon this capital thriftily for a long, monotonous, uneventful existence. Or, on the other hand, you can spend it lavishly in a stressful, intense, but perhaps more colorful and exciting life.

Adapting yourself
to what you are

The choice is not always yours. After all, you had little control over what happened to you as a child. You have had little control over many environmental aspects of your life. You have had no control over the hereditary facets of your personality. You may think that you have the potential to become President, or a great artist, or perhaps a leader in the business world—and you may feel that only a lack of opportunity or "bad luck" or perhaps your own culpable laziness kept you from scaling the heights. This is not so, however. If you have

been lucky enough to find a pleasing social environment, the job that makes you happy, and the life partner
who will enable you to live at an ideal pace, then you
must realize that you are the recipient of a great deal of
good fortune and that you will be comparatively
healthy and happy no matter what your wealth and
social position.

What you have in you must come out; otherwise you
might explode at the wrong places or become hope-
lessly hemmed in by frustrations. It has been said that
the great art is to express your vitality through the particular channels and at the particular speed for which
nature has endowed you. If a man's store of adaptive
energy is small and if he is forced by life into a position
where he must work hard and stressfully, he will undoubtedly lead a short and unhappy life. On the other
hand, with a great deal of adaptive energy, and the opportunity of working under less stressful conditions, life
should be comparatively long and happy.

If you find yourself tied to a small and monotonous
job, you are bound to explode at the wrong places.
These explosions can take many forms. You may become an angry, bitter person; you may become frustrated and suffer physical and mental breakdown; you
may take to drink, or to crime, or to some other anti-
social behavior.

Of course, it does not all depend upon the amount of
adaptive energy you are given at birth and the circumstances in which you find yourself beyond that time.

158

You can alter your lot or improve it. However, that which you are able to do must be done within the limits of what is physically possible for you. Your adaptive energy is like a bank account that you use up by making withdrawals but that you can never increase by making deposits. Unfortunately, the solution is not to just stop withdrawing—that would mean the end of life. Nor is the solution to withdraw just enough for survival—that would mean a life of vegetation that would be worse, inevitably, than death. The intelligent answer is to withdraw generously but never to squander.

Emotionally induced
physical ailments

Improper mental states can cause trouble in your physical make-up. Fifty per cent of all people who seek medical attention have been found to suffer from ailments that have been brought about or made worse by such emotional factors as prolonged worry, anxiety, or fear. In fact, out of one thousand diseases described in a textbook of medicine, it is said that emotionally induced illness is as common as all the other nine hundred ninety-nine put together. How you think has a definite effect on how you feel. You translate your woes from the language of the mind to the language of the body. Whatever you allow to affect your mind in the way of pain or pleasure, hope or fear, will extend its influence to your heart. Financial worries, a monotonous job, strain at the office, emotional upsets in the home—these and many more may show themselves physically as digestive ailments, skin disorders, headaches, allergies and high blood pressure. You cannot go into a drugstore, however, and buy a bottle of psychosomatic medicine. The first thing to do when you feel unwell is to have your doctor give you a thorough checkup. He will learn from his tests and your answers to his questions whether there is something organically wrong and how much of your illness is derived from emotional sources. Finding the cause is the first step on the way to finding the cure.

And the cause, it appears, seems to lie in the mad scramble of everyday living. The exasperations of each day get you keyed up. The tension accompanies you home and keeps you awake—unless you have worked out for yourself an effective way of releasing it. One evil result of your hasty living is that so often you fail to solve your problems adequately. The result is a state of anxiety. It is wholesome to have fear when that fear is an alarm, a warning of impending danger. Unfortunately, too many people go around in a perpetual state of anxiety which prevents them from relaxing and keeps them tense. The protective patterns set in motion by their bodies are overworked.

The best executives have moments of doubt and weariness, but they rise from their depression by returning to principles they have learned. One of life's most health-giving virtues is the ability to meet disappointment and frustration well. An angry outburst is a poor response to disappointment, because it heals nothing, because it replaces nothing of what has been lost, and because it takes its toll on the body. An angry man is not one who is doing something, but one who is suffering something to be done to him. He is permitting his dignity to be lowered. And, as if that were not bad enough, he is also interfering with his digestion, disrupting his circulation, and putting undue strain on his body's defensive organisms.

Some people, to avoid being disappointed after something happens, try to forestall events. They wrench them out of their place in the future and worry about them today. It is as though worry becomes interest paid on trouble before it falls due. Elizabeth Barrett Browning in one of her poems defined worry eloquently when she said that it is with us when, "We walk upon the shadow of hills across a level thrown, and pant like climbers."

Chronic worry

brings on fatigue

In extreme cases, worry turns into what is called "doubting folly," in which you doubt whether you can

trust your own senses. You forever find yourself returning to see if you have locked a door, or rereading a letter
time and again to make sure you have expressed yourself properly, or wondering all through the evening
whether you have told your secretary about an important appointment the next day.

While textbooks on psychosomatic medicine list
many kinds of illness that chronic worry can bring on,
the most common is fatigue of one sort or another.
There is nothing dramatic about fatigue—as there is
about dyspepsia or ulcers or arthritis. It just creeps upon
you, seeping through your body like poison. You can
consult a competent physician who will tell you that
you have no sign of tuberculosis, or heart trouble, or
any other demonstrable disease. There will be nothing
wrong with your body machinery, but you still will feel
tired. You get your wires crossed, and the wrong mes-
sages come through to the brain.

Boredom sets up stresses that give you feelings of
fatigue. Long hours at your desk, repeated day after
day, result in muscular tension that can be more physically fatiguing than heavy manual labor. The boredom
of a woman's endlessly repetitive work sets up the same
kind of stresses. The housewife's day is a series of minor
crises that, when added to her jam-packed schedule,
bring on unhealthy amounts of tension.

Tension is an insidious thing. You have what you
would call "one of those days," and tension suddenly
erupts. You have become a victim of miserable head-

ache, taut nerves and muscles, a queasy stomach. Fatigue can even be brought on by too much conversation. Energy is often wasted in unnecessary speech.

Are there any signs that indicate to you that your tension-level has built up to the point of breaking? Perhaps you'll recognize some of these:

A loss of interest in people, work, play, and hobbies that used to fascinate you;

Uncontrollable anger at inanimate objects like a stuck zipper, a dead battery, a blown fuse;

Complete inability to make a decision with the result of so much unfinished work that you cannot possibly make up your mind where to begin;

Chronic fatigue, with no great physical exertion to account for it;

Discovery that you are pressing so hard—in business, in human relationships, in ambitions—that you are missing too many shots.

Make worry

work for you

Stresses develop in every area of life. Unless you're endowed with nerves of steel, with executive ability, or with great intelligence, you have to learn to live within your abilities. In other words, you must steer clear of stress—unless you can take it. Otherwise you will find yourself a readily acceptable member of the "coronary club."

There is no purpose in being a supercharged worrier. But if you are, then there is only one thing to do with the worrying habit: Put it on a constructive, rather than a destructive, circuit. If you properly harness the energy that your anxiety produces, you could well be a potential dynamo. When you begin to worry, determine what it is that is making you worry. This may take real effort, since failure to recognize a specific problem is a major cause of bewildering anxiety. But looking your problem in the face may show it up as an illusion, and it will either vanish by itself or it will emerge clearly without any emotional fuzziness. Once you have pinpointed the problem, list the possible solutions to it. Then go over the list carefully and choose the one that applies most specifically. Develop a plan of action— and carry it out. If you don't do this, you'll get right back into the worry whirlpool. There is a great futility about worrying since most of the things you worry about are things that actually never happen. These are the wasted worries. But far more dangerous is the effect that your worries have on your health. Think of worry in its original definition—that is, "to strangle or to choke." That is actually what worry does to you. It strangles or it chokes—not only your thinking, but your emotions and your state of health.

Overwork is often accused of being the cause of mental and physical illness. However, this reason was given so often by patients that medical researchers made a study of overwork as it related to such illness. The results were rather startling simply because it was discovered that work itself was rarely a cause. What the study did uncover most frequently was that unsatisfactory relationships with a supervisor and rigid, self-driving attitudes were the problem. Of the group of patients studied, less than ten per cent showed symptoms of illness that could be directly attributed to their work. The others revealed in interviews that conflicts with fellow employees, illness in a co-worker with the same type of job, or a pre-existing state of tension which made the patient assume an undue load of responsibilities and obligations, were the direct causes.

The road of life is crowded with traffic and you must accept its conditions and drive on. You cannot expect that the world will allow you to carry a "learner's permit" and have an "instructor" sitting beside you all the time. The road you travel is often a dangerous one— but you must keep your head and know where you are going. The moment you hesitate, you begin to worry. The moment you begin to worry, you set up a pattern of high-tension terrors that will slowly deplete the balance in your adaptive-energy bank account.

14

Avoiding Occupational Stress

A great deal of interest is being shown these days in the health of working people, both in factories and in offices. It is a recognized fact that if unhappiness exists— either physical or mental—work suffers, accidents in the industrial plants increase, and jobs are jeopardized. This type of liability exists not only for the employee, but also for the top executive. The unhappy executive may become less creative in his work or he may even fail in an important project when an outstanding job has been expected of him.

The stresses associated with the management of a business—just as much as those related to the management of a classroom or a home—can have a definite effect upon health. Much as an employee may have his doubts about it, leadership has its price. But its toll can be cut down. The inescapable characteristic of the executive job is its tyrannical demands in terms of time and continuous mental and physical pressure. The difficulty is that the "top man" can never escape responsibility. Decisions he must make expose him to frequent emotional stress. His administrative duties build tension. But if an executive does nothing about the stresses and tensions under which he works, then he becomes as much a problem to his organization as the employee on the production line with emotional problems.

The executive is, of course, a man who has risen because of his ability to cope with more than one problem at a time. He is a man not content with keeping his belt in the same notch it was in five years earlier. But something more is needed if a man is to maintain his equanimity in a world full of stress. The executive's ability is really tested only when he has to lead his company or his department under unusual strain. That demands the inner calm that follows a frank facing of difficulty and fear and disappointment, and even the prospect of disaster. But the good executive must ease the pressure on himself by admitting the impossibility of being a success by every standard, of always being right, of never suffering a setback. Too many tensions are the result of trying to act like a superman. If you don't mind admitting your failures, you can conserve your power. You will suffer injury once in a while, but you will recuperate because of a reserve of unused strength. The best balanced people are not obsessively devoted to their jobs. They have a natural rhythm in work and rest, an answer in part at least to the stress of living.

Many industries are investigating work failures among their employees with the expectation of finding some relievable background of trouble in the lives of these people to explain the decreases, sudden or gradual, in their efficiency. The investigations often do reveal unhappy or worrisome situations in their private lives for which guidance from a sympathetic manager or an understanding industrial nurse or psychiatrist is often available and effective.

Sometimes just a sympathetic listener—where none has been expected—and an opportunity to tell his troubles, to "ventilate," will do a great deal toward the improvement of the individual's outlook and work performance. Deep-seated, unrevealed troubles often cause not only unhappiness in the person involved but, by a sort of contagious process, may involve his fellow workers or employees to a degree that the success of an entire project is jeopardized.

Occupational stress and unhappiness

Happiness in work radiates just as effectively for success as unhappiness does for failure. One person in an organization can spoil the morale of the entire enterprise. This does not mean that inexcusable inefficiency or neglect of work can be condoned in any field of endeavor, however. What it does mean is that when an individual who normally has done good work suddenly or gradually declines in efficiency, the cause should be sympathetically looked for before a sentence of dismissal is pronounced.

Just as occupational stress has been found to be a vital factor in the breakdown of emotional happiness, so it has been found to be one of the most significant factors in the occurrence of coronary heart disease. In a series of studies done recently, it was found that certain specific situations pertained among those men who suffered heart attacks under circumstances that seemed to be directly related to their jobs. These situations were:

A full-time job during the day and a second job in the evening;

169

A work period of sixty hours or more a week in the period which immediately preceded the heart attack;

Unusual fear, insecurity, discontent, frustration, or inadequacy with respect to their employment.

This study, which was made by Dr. Henry I. Russek and Dr. Burton L. Zohman, investigated the three chief causes to which heart attacks have been attributed: a family history of heart disease, addiction to high-fat foods, and occupational stress. In the case of a family history of heart disease, it was found that in one hundred cases of coronary patients and one hundred healthy people (whose ages were similar, as well as their jobs and ethnic origins), sixty-seven per cent of the coronaries had family histories of heart disease but so did forty per cent of the healthy patients. Among the same test groups, it was found that fifty-three per cent of the coronary patients often ate high-fat foods but so did twenty per cent of the healthy patients. The startling factor of the research was that ninety-one per cent of the heart patients suffered from acute job stress while only twenty per cent of the healthy people did. It was obvious that occupational stress was the most critical factor.

The conclusion that these two medical researchers came to was that severe and unrelieved occupational stress is the key to identifying candidates to early coronary heart disease. This did not necessarily mean that stress was the only factor affecting coronary arterial disease. But the guilty finger pointed doubly when it was found that an excess of cholesterol in the blood stream was also associated with these attacks and that occupational stress actually did affect the amount of cholesterol which was being deposited in the arteries. Other researchers, working in other areas, found results that bore out this study. Among the Navajo Indians and among the Eskimos—two civilizations in which stress as we understand it is at a minimum—coronary artery disease was found to be rare, and this despite the fact that the diets of both civilizations are high in fat. Studies in South Africa discovered that increased job responsibilities went hand in hand with a higher rate of coronary artery disease.

Other studies indicated quite clearly that the susceptibility to coronary disease must be due to something other than diet. And since stress increased the cholesterol content in the blood, again a finger was pointed in the direction of this new-found enemy.

*The four steps
to heart attack*

As you have already read, occupational stress is translated into a coronary attack through four simple steps. First, the stress affects the endocrine system, especially

171

the adrenal glands. Then, the hormone balance and fat-metabolism are disturbed, producing excessively high blood cholesterol. Thirdly, the cholesterol is deposited in the arteries, causing atherosclerosis. Fourthly, this narrowing of the arteries creates conditions for coronary heart attack.

Occupational stress is, however, not a one-time thing. It is a continuous and cumulative process. Physical strain is often present, but it is accompanied by strong mental and emotional stress as well. A ditchdigger rarely has a coronary heart attack because physical work is readily compensated for by food and sleep. But men under occupational stress who are straining to keep up with the rest of society and with the Joneses, who are straining to conform with convention and to get ahead, these are the ones who are the more likely sufferers of coronary heart attack. Among such a group you will find insurance salesmen who work evenings to get extra business after having worked all day, foremen who are under pressure from the management to produce more but also under pressure from the men to be "a good guy," and a man who does piecework and who has a hard time making ends meet and therefore pushes himself. You can probably add many more categories to that listing. But making a long list of occupations in which occupational stress can be excessive and therefore deadly is not going to solve the problem. The problem can only be solved by curbing and reducing stress.

The problem can only be solved by adopting a life pattern which balances work and play, exercise and rest.

Of course the most important thing you should do if you feel you may be under stress, or are fatigued and run down, is to have an examination by your physician. The physician today does not look only for organic disease. He also tries to seek the cause of unfitness in social and personal factors. Above all, do not try self-medication. There are many dangers which present themselves in the unscientific use of tranquilizing drugs. People do not react in the same way to pills that relieve stress. Some become depressed or develop psychoneurotic difficulties. Others feel so free of pain that they fail to take necessary medical measures. Others are so energized that they neglect to take proper rest.

There's less room at the top

The next step is to recognize certain basic factors that exist in your relationship with your job. In the first place, it is vital that you eliminate the incessant striving on your job. The desire to get ahead is commendable. But there are limitations which are built in within you. There is just so much that you can do, just so much pressure that you can put yourself under. In other words, there is a point of maximum effort—and you must recognize that point. Beyond it, you are accomplishing nothing more. Instead, you are only forcing your system into stressful situations that will bring about great damage.

Secondly, eliminate from your thinking the false sense of hurry which does not necessarily make for greater efficiency. Speed and efficiency are not synonymous. Find your own level of working speed. Beyond that level, you are going to find that your capacity for mistakes will increase. Not only are you then working at a level of lesser efficiency, but you are setting up within yourself a series of stresses from the moment you recognize that your productivity is slipping in efficiency.

Thirdly, be satisfied with your job. It is all very well to want to be the boss, but if this is a position that you can never reach, you are establishing for yourself anxieties and tensions from which you may never recover. You see, it is not the man who knows his own capacities who suffers so much from stress as the employee who wants desperately to be the boss but can never make it, who sets his goal far beyond his ability.

There is no doubt that the modern business organization can lead to increases of stress because it is so big and complex. There is less room at the top and there is a growing need for subordinates. Besides, what's wrong with being *second* vice-president? You can't all be first!

Industry has come to recognize that a man can only

do so much. Now it is up to you to recognize just how much you can do—and not attempt to do more. The pace that you set must be within the reasonable capacity of both your physical and emotional selves. Assuredly, the end result will be the same production—and probably even better.

15

Relieving Occupational Stress

It goes without saying that good work conditions contribute to physical and mental well-being. Therefore, it is a natural conclusion that good work conditions can help ease the tensions of your job. Your ability to relax is one of the surest symptoms of your mental health. After you have been keyed up to accomplish a task, you have to slacken off instead of whipping yourself into further exertion. If you relax away the little tensions as they occur, you stand a very good chance of preventing the accumulation of big tensions. Every person, however, must find out what his own needs are in the way of relaxation, just as everyone needs to estimate his own needs in the way of sleep. It is important, nevertheless, not to become strenuously relaxed. Dr. Selye has warned, for instance, that a vacation in Florida may not be the right thing for a busy executive. "Activity may be this man's way of relieving pressure," he said. "He may build up more internal pressure idling than if he were at work."

While the whole stress concept may seem new to you, actually your grandfather's doctor may have given him advice a half-century ago that your doctor would give you today. It was not uncommon for medical men to tell an overworked man at the turn of the century that for his heart's sake he should diminish his pace and obtain the benefits of some proper relaxation.

How can you ease the tensions on your job? The most important piece of advice is to get plenty of rest, simply because you have to compensate for the physical activity and the emotional strain of the job. Sleep, then, is a vital factor and you have already learned of its importance and of its need.

But next to sleep, there is the problem of long hours at a desk, repeated day after day. Such a work pattern results in muscular tension that can be more physically fatiguing than heavy manual labor. It is not overwork that makes the typical "tired executive" tired. It is tension caused by lack of exercise. Where, however, can the busy executive find time for pushups and deep knee-bends? The answer is simply that he does not have to. Anyone can keep in shape at his office desk by making a few simple exercises part of his daily routine. And since twice as many sedentary people as active people have heart attacks every year, it is obvious why exercise should be looked to as a prime means of easing the tensions of your job. Not that it is a total answer, but in almost every case it is a big part of the answer.

The law of
flight or fight

From the physiological point of view, all men are animals. They are, therefore, subject to Cannon's Law of Flight or Fight, which states simply that an animal will either run or he will fight when irritated. The irritation, however, need not be of a physical nature. As a businessman your system goes through the same kind of changes as a frightened bear, for instance, when you are stimulated by irritation or by a problem. The difficulty for you is that you cannot release your tensions in the same way as the bear will; he will either run or he will stand on his hind legs and fight back.

Let us say for instance that you get a particularly irritating memo from another department in the office.

You get mad and you become tense. You would like to take the elevator down to the man in the other department and punch him in the nose. But you can't—in fact, you cannot even reveal that you would like to do this. Moreover, you probably won't even bark at your secretary or show any signs of anger in the office—it isn't the thing to do. Therefore the tension that has been caused by this memo cannot be released. The tension will soon back up into a headache or a backache or an upset stomach. It will set into motion the General Adaptation Syndrome—stress—and dependent upon how continuous the stress remains due to other irritating situations is your emotional and physiological well-being.

To keep operating at your maximum efficiency, you should learn how to dispel tension before it has a chance to build up and cause damage. Usually the tension is localized in the muscles of the neck and shoulders and back, as you have already learned. The trick is, then, to loosen these muscles before they become too tight. There are some very simple ways to do this—and thus prevent the tension from building.

1. Shrug your shoulders several times every time you perform a routine action such as hanging up the telephone, opening a drawer, or signing a letter.

2. Every time you sit down, take a deep breath and exhale slowly.

3. At least once every thirty minutes, lean back in your chair and stretch all your muscles quite hard.

4. Every time you go through the door of your office, place your hands on the opposite sides of the doorway and push sideways as though you were trying to push down the doorposts.

5. Every time you get up from your chair, bend down and try to touch your toes, letting your arms and shoulders fall loosely.

If you do these things regularly, they will become secondary reflexes and your muscles will unconsciously learn how to untense in tense situations.

Ordinary ways
of exercising

You are probably laughing to yourself right now and asking: "How can I do this in the office without looking silly?" The answer is that once the other people in the office realize what you are doing, you will probably convince them that they should all be doing it. Nobody is going to think it silly once they realize that you have discovered the secret of combating death-dealing tensions. Nobody is going to think it silly once they realize that you have learned how to avoid high-tension terrors. The only way to fight tension and fatigue is to get your muscles in condition to withstand the strain of your job. Once you realize that you can exercise all day long in the normal course of your business, you will find many ways of working exercise into your daily pattern. It will do wonders for you. The best thing about it is that it is easy.

For instance, on your way to work in the morning, do you do any walking at all? Or does your wife drive you straight to the railroad station and do you take a cab from the station to the office? Why not try walking at one end or the other, and if the distance is too far at either end make sure that you walk part of the way, at least a quarter mile. Or if you live in the city and take the bus to work, why not get off four or five blocks from your stop and walk the rest of the way—whether it rains, snows or sleets.

What about using the stairs in your office building at least once a day. Of course, if you work on the sixteenth floor, you shouldn't walk up all the way, but you can take the elevator to the fifteenth floor and walk up the last flight on your way in every morning. And when you leave in the evening, unless you happen to work on a high floor of a skyscraper, why not try walking down the stairs. Walking down is hardly any physical strain— and it is good exercise.

Have you ever tried office-chair pushups? Put your hands on the arms of your chair and lift your body half a dozen times. This will use up the extra adrenalin in your system and will cause your muscles to return to normal.

Most important, how much time do you take for lunch? Most employees have forty-five minutes or an hour. Too many busy executives, however, rush through their meals in twenty minutes and then wonder why they get indigestion. You probably have a favorite restaurant within a few hundred yards of the office. Why not find one four or five blocks away and walk to it several times a week. After lunch, walk leisurely back to the office. Window shop, look at the pretty girls. Above all, try to avoid using the restaurant as a second office—don't make business luncheon appointments unless they are absolutely necessary.

The same principle should apply to traveling to and from the office. Train yourself to keep business out of your mind until the moment you are ready to start your day. This is very difficult to do sometimes, but it is quite possible if you do it consciously. You then save about one and a half hours wastage of nervous energy every day. And when you finally leave the office for the day, try putting business behind you. Leave it at your desk rather than taking it home with you. You cannot overcome the stresses of the job if you take the worries it entails to bed with you. You must keep abreast of things in your work and take it seriously. But no man can keep his mind focused constantly on one subject with impunity. Change of thought is needed for mental relaxation. You cannot afford to go through the financial pages of your newspaper at breakfast and then spend hours at various trade journals when you are at home in the evening.

Change your job
or change your position

What about your working conditions? If they are good they contribute to physical and mental well-being. Efficiency can be increased and errors reduced, as well as absenteeism lowered, if the noise level in your office is decreased. Comfort, ability and health are added to by adequate ventilation assuring a sufficient supply of oxygen. Proper lighting contributes its share.

And suppose you do not like your job, suppose it doesn't give you real pleasure? How much more tired you are at the end of the day with job-dislike as a contributing factor! It may be necessary to change your employment—this is something to be seriously considered.

However, while some people may find it necessary to change their job, countless thousands can improve their health by just changing their *position*. Stress in one area may be relieved by shifting part of the load to another area, as when the man who is so unfortunate as to have to carry home a heavily laden briefcase shifts it from hand to hand. To walk around your office or home at intervals is a break that relieves physical and mental

183

stress. There was a great deal of stress-release value in the old rocking chair. Do not accept hurry and tension as unavoidable. Do not allow yourself to be pressed down by the sheer weight of things to do.

Too many men and women exceed what is necessary. They are not content to be eminent, but compromise their victories by extra effort. Success incites them to greater activity and more urgent endeavor. The only solution they know for their mounting need of self-expression is to work harder and harder. They become tense and anxiety-ridden. They burn themselves out. That picture is all too common. Yet the very men who are putting so great a strain on their physical capacities know very well that it is in moments of relaxed and easy work that they are most efficient; that their most rewarding successes are scored when, having determined upon a course of action, they unclamp their intellectual and physical machinery and let it run free.

16

Stress in Play

Inevitably it is you who can make the most important contribution toward your own good health. It is Dr. Selye's contention that to do this you must discover your own best stress level and make every effort to live at that level. What is your best stress level? It is the point at which the stresses that affect you have not built to the point of excessive expenditure, nor have they failed to reach the point of generous, though controlled, usage.

You have already seen how stress can often be the spice of life as well as how, on the other hand, it may have damaging side effects that can shorten life. Since all normal living can cause wear and tear on the body, a game of golf, a game of badminton, even a chess match, can exert stress upon you just as much as shoveling, or a fit of anger, or a day at the office.

A little less than one-third of your life is spent in doing your daily labors—whether you dig ditches, keep books, practice law, are a housekeeper, or teach school. About one-third of your life is spent in the process of replenishing your energies—and, under ideal conditions, easing the tensions for the day that follows—in sleep. The remainder, a little more than one-third of your life, is supposed to be spent in recreation, social activity, amusement, social obligation. Just what portion of that time is spent in some form of "play" depends upon you. Equally does the amount of stress—good or bad—that is developed during that play time depend upon you.

There is an old saying that all work and no play makes Jack a dull boy. And there is a newer joke that all work and no play makes "jack"—especially for the person who thinks of life as having only a financial purpose. But work has to be balanced with play. The proverb about Jack being a dull boy if all he does is work still makes sense. In addition, all work may also give Jack an ulcer or, worse still, lead him onto the path to heart disease. The difficulty for most Jacks—and Jills—is that they have trouble taking it easy for a long enough time to get some fun out of life. They have not learned the basic rule that just as work time must be scheduled, so must time for recreation be scheduled.

Get some fun

out of life

It all boils down to a simple formula: *Get some fun out of life!* This is one of the surest ways of handling your tension successfully and weathering the rough spots of life more smoothly. On the other hand, don't schedule yourself into an excess of entertainment. Don't set up a routine where you *must* go bowling on Mondays, and play cards on Wednesdays, and take in a double feature at the movie house on Saturday nights. This kind of compulsive leisure activity leads only to stress again. In this way, you do things under stress because everyone else is doing them.

Let your entertainment be more of a do-it-as-the-spirit-moves-you kind of fun. Of course, you may have certain responsibilities that don't permit you to be so devil-may-care at all times. Perhaps you can't suddenly go off to the movies with your wife because there is no baby sitter available at the last moment. Maybe the Smiths can't come over to play cards when the whim occurs to you at 7:30 P.M., because they have other arrangements for the evening. But just as long as your desires for recreation don't become compulsive, then a hitch in your plans can't become stressful.

Just as work can occasionally be a kind of cure for emotional situations that are hard to bear—such as the death of a loved one, a divorce, or the breaking of an engagement—so play can be a cure for the emotional tensions that build up during work. The same formula is involved. The easiest way to stop stewing about your troubles is to get busy at something else. That "something else" can be an interesting hobby, one which can be relaxing as well as constructive, one which will keep you interested beyond just a week, or a month, or a year. Your rest has to be coupled with leisurely leisure, and an absorbing hobby will often do the trick. It might be golf, it might be painting, or gardening or astronomy. Perhaps you want to take up collecting—stamps, or coins, or anything that will open new frontiers of excitement, education, and emotional relief from tension.

Above all, however, you must slow the pace of your leisure—it must be leisurely. You must make your home a place to which you can come for relaxation. Make your home the kind of home your parents had, one in which there was singing, and dancing, and conversation, and reading. Home should not be just a stopping-over point between your business day and your social day. If you become heavily committed with social activities, your evening meal will be rushed, the time you spend with

188

your wife and children will shrink to a trickle, and before you know it the stress level within you will be built to the point of breaking. It all boils down to an ability to say "no." You must say it to yourself and you must say it to others. You must learn to use it lest you find yourself on a social treadmill the pace of which can be twice as killing as the work treadmill on which you are forced to run from nine to five daily.

Recreation can be destructive, too

Be warned that your social life can become burdensome hard work once it reaches the point where you would rather "get out" of the entertaining and the flitting-about that you have imposed upon yourself. Do not let your recreation become more destructive than your work. Make sure that you are not entertaining primarily for business reasons. Make sure that you are not entertaining primarily as a way of social climbing. Don't try to "keep up with the Joneses" in the social whirl. Make sure that your week-ends are restful so that you can tackle the business stresses of the week that follows.

Spend your leisure time with people whom you enjoy and who can relax you. Arrange your free time in such a way so that there will be times that you can go for a

walk alone, enabling yourself to reflect. Look upon social activity as a form of mental and physical relaxation.
Above all, do not go running off on a last-minute invitation if your plans had already called for a quiet evening at home or a visit to the movies with your wife.
Remember how to say "no."

Wise use of your leisure holds the germ of survival
in this complicated civilization of ours. Play, fun, and
laughter, all of these are agents of health. They can
promote good digestion, they can soothe your nerves,
they can stimulate your circulation, they can give power
to your heart—and they can ward off the feeling of old
age. Your leisure time is a time to stretch your limbs
and to let go of your tensions. It is a time to laugh and to
be cheerful.

It was William James who, in a lecture entitled "The
Gospel of Relaxation," said that "The sovereign vol-
untary path to cheerfulness, if our spontaneous cheerfulness be lost, is to sit up cheerfully, to look around
cheerfully, and to act and speak as if cheerfulness were
already there." Try smiling, try laughing! See how
quickly a big smile seems to loosen the inner muscles
that are the first to tense up—for instance, those muscles
in and around your stomach. See how quickly laughing
will become an unconscious reaction when you suddenly realize that something has happened over which
you have no control. You must be able to ignore situations of this sort, and laughing at them is your best de-

fense against them. It is important to remember that the difference between play and work has nothing to do with the nature of the activity. For instance, farming is a job if you follow it as a living. However, if you dig in your garden on week-ends as a change from your workaday job the rest of the week, it is a form of play. By the same token, entertaining friends occasionally is fun. But a woman who has to entertain frequently, because she feels her husband's business or profession requires it, is carrying out a duty so that after a while it becomes more of a chore than a pleasure. The man who carries a mailbag during work hours as a postman finds that his many miles of walking are a job. But on his day off, if he were to put a knapsack on his back and go for a leisurely hike in the country, he would be playing. It's the old story of the busman's holiday. Does that mean that if you enjoy your work you can make it serve for play as well? It has been done—by such men as Thomas Edison. But few of you are Edisons able to live to work instead of working to live and suffer no harm for it. Cervantes wrote that "The bow cannot always stand bent, nor can human frailties subsist without some lawful recreation." With the pressure-cooker existence that most people lead today that is doubly true.

Above all, do not handicap yourself with the attitude that you have no capacity, or ability, or talent for one or another thing. There are countless thousands of people who have shown remarkable ability that they never realized they had. Try to find at least one activity that you can be good at—but not necessarily at which you must excel. If you have any pride in performance, you will try to be as good as your potential will permit. But don't forget that second best has its satisfactions, too. Bear in mind that your play needs are not fixed. They vary with changing circumstances and available energies. As an adolescent you went along with the crowd. In early adulthood you leaned heavily toward recreations that would help you in your social life or in getting along in your work. Now you must take a closer look at your play needs and consider as well the needs of your mate and of the other members of your family. You have to find a design for play that is flexible enough to be altered to accord with changing requirements— whether physical, mental, or emotional.

Leisure is one of your most precious and personal possessions. It is the best antidote against harmful stresses. Therefore, let it work *for* you instead of *against* you. Learn how really to enjoy it.

17

Growing Old Healthily

That hurry and worry do more to speed the process of aging than any other factor has been emphasized in every chapter of this book.

It has been shown that worry and tension lead to stress, and that stress is more fatiguing and consumes more energy than the hardest kind of physical labor. Stress also produces extreme imbalances in the body's system so that the proper blood circulation is impaired and as a result the heart can be easily damaged.

It may sound trite, therefore, to say: Stop worrying

and take things easier. But all the evidence you have read indicates that there is no simpler or more effective way of adding years to your life. In other words, if you take your time, you will have more of it!

It goes without saying that you *want* to live longer. In order to accomplish this, therefore, you must dispense with worry and hurry. You must utilize the formula you learned earlier: *Take it easy!*

The scientific investigations that you have read about in these pages have shown you incontrovertibly that hyperactive people tend to be much shorter lived than easygoing people whose energy output is moderate and well balanced. You undoubtedly all know of someone who, though there seemed to be no reason for him to suddenly collapse, died in the prime of life. Usually these people are of the human-dynamo type. They are the kind who generate and use up energy—who squander it—at a terrific rate. They are the kind who are seldom still for a minute. In fact, you sometimes wonder if they even sleep restfully. They seem to thrive on living at this pace. But when they reach their prime, the supply of life energy has exhausted itself—and they become just another mortality statistic.

And while it is sound advice not to waste and dissipate your energies, it is equally as sound not to go to the other extreme and embrace laziness. After all, what you accomplish with your life is more important than how long it is. In addition, scientific research has found

194

that you are likely to live longer if you do well whatever you are doing. For example, if you are a successful housewife and mother, the odds are that you will have a longer life span than if you have made a fizzle of the job. A study of some ten thousand notably successful persons in eighteen countries showed that a vast majority of them averaged much longer life spans than their fellow man. The researchers could conclude only that their longevity was significantly related to their occupational happiness and resulting eminence.

But this does not mean that you should drive yourself or overtax yourself either mentally or physically. This will shorten your life. Furthermore, it is not necessary. You can be just as successful if you take things in your stride. Tests have shown that any problem can be solved more quickly and more easily when you are mentally and physically relaxed.

Six steps to
a longer life

There are some very definite ways in which you can learn to relax in everyday life. These rules will help you handle your tensions more successfully and weather the rough spots of life more smoothly. They will help you in much the same fashion as a stabilizer on a big passenger ship—acting as a leveling influence despite the storm-tossed waves that you must travel through.

What are these ways that will help you live longer without the taxation of stress?

First, and perhaps most important, *make sure that you have a regular medical checkup*. The regularity of such a periodic checkup is almost as important as the checkup itself. It is useless going to your doctor next week, and then not seeing him again for three years. It is quite as useless as doing the same thing with your dentist. It is quite as useless as doing the same thing with your car. There has to be an established regularity with which these checkups take place. Ask your doctor when he would like to see you next. He may say six months, he may say more frequently, or he may say less frequently. But whatever it is, make sure that you do keep a close check on your physical condition. Just as your mind can affect your body's working order, so your physical condition can affect your outlook on life. If you keep yourself physically fit, you will have more zest for living and you will be able to take stress and handle tensions more easily.

Second, *try balancing work with play* in a better fashion than you have—if, indeed, you have balanced these two aspects of your waking hours. Try getting some fun out of life. Just because you have reached your middle years does not mean to say that you should stop exercising. This is the secret of so many former champions of sport. In virtually every field—be it tennis or golf, boxing or baseball—you will find that

196

former "greats" are still in wonderful physical condition. Their secret is continued exercise. If you are not finding enough time for recreation, then perhaps you ought to re-schedule your time to make room for a little re-creating. Without it, the result might be wreck-creating. Remember that an interesting hobby can be just as relaxing as physical activity—and it can be constructive as well. Whatever it is you choose for recreation, however, make sure it is something you are going to enjoy. Don't choose a field of activity simply so that you can say you are finding recreation. It won't be long before recreation of that kind will begin to destroy you with boredom. Remember, too, that in balancing your work with play, work can occasionally be a kind of cure for emotional situations that are hard to bear. If you are the kind of person who does not stop stewing about your troubles, it may help at times to get busy at some job or other.

Third, *learn to get your troubles off your chest*. Psychologists and psychiatrists call this "ventilating." You sort of open the windows and let the stale air blow out and the fresh air blow in. You will be surprised how relaxed you feel, how your tensions quickly ease, when you talk out your troubles with a sympathetic friend. And if you feel that your worries are too serious to confide to a sympathetic friend, and if a problem begins to get you down, why not discuss it with your family doctor or your own religious advisor. You may even find some understanding member of your own family, often your own mate, with whom you can talk out your problem. Don't expect answers, or solutions, or panaceas for your problems. But you can expect a lightening of the burden—for often the burden is made twice as heavy due to the fact that you find it difficult to talk about it. Sometimes the person you talk to can help you get your feelings into focus. Just the open expression of your feelings may help you see your problems in a new light.

Fourth, when you get upset or angry, *try "blowing off steam."* You will be surprised how effective opening the "safety valve" can be toward working off your tensions. In one explosive outburst you can sometimes relieve the massive accumulation of stresses that you have built up over hours, or days, or sometimes weeks. Blowing off steam does not necessarily mean that you have to punch someone in the nose. Why not pick up a pillow and give it a good wallop? Or put your coat on and take a long walk at a brisk pace? Perhaps you want to run around the block a few times? Look at yourself in the mirror and imagine how ridiculous the situation has become in the light of what you will think of it ten years from now—laugh at yourself, heartily and long. Perhaps singing at the top of your lungs, or shouting your head off—or even a good cry—until you are exhausted will prevent the stresses that can produce chronic illness and inevitably chronic unhappiness. Maybe you will feel better pitching into some activity, like working in the garden or taking in a round of golf. Any of these things will not only help to relieve anger, but will make it easier to face and handle irritating problems more calmly. It is infinitely better to exhaust yourself in this way than to stew and steam and settle yourself down into a rut of irritability and accumulative stresses.

Fifth, *recognize the fact that certain situations cannot be changed*. There are circumstances that are beyond your control. Unfortunately, too many people become upset by such circumstances. They feel that everything should be within their control. They get the childhood feeling of omnipotence and desire to change all things to a mold that they feel best. Sometimes people feel that they should try to change other people, make them over to suit their own ideals. Then, when they find that this cannot be done, they feel frustrated or let down. If, however, you can learn to accept those things which cannot be changed, if you can learn to look for the best in other people—and recognize that nobody, least of all yourself, is faultless—then you can overcome one of the major areas of stress-giving frustration.

Sixth, *try well-placed procrastination.* In other words, try loafing from time to time, try putting things off until tomorrow, or even try getting away from it all for a short time. Very active people who feel guilty about occasionally just sitting and doing plain nothing should give themselves a chance to learn the art of loafing. Of course, there is an extreme. Too much inactivity will bring boredom. Boredom will, in turn, cause stress. But a few minutes every day of doing just nothing may help you tackle your work with renewed enthusiasm. Sometimes it is important to just let some things go. When a workload seems overwhelming, remember the physical limitations of working. You can only do one thing at a time. Therefore, concentrate on the particular job at hand. Or set yourself about doing the most important of the tasks that face you. Then, when the first job is finished, go on to a subsequent one. And stop worrying about everything that is yet to be done. Stop worrying about the things that you can set aside until later. There are always things that can be put off until tomorrow. And work usually goes faster and smoother when you have this attitude of doing one thing at a time. When your job, or a problem, makes you feel that you are going around in circles, divert yourself. Step off the treadmill. It may be as simple a thing as going to the movies, or picking up a magazine and reading for a while. Or it may be a visit to a friend. Whatever it is, it will help you get out of the rut you have gotten yourself in. Remember that there is never any harm in running away from a painful situation just long enough to catch your breath and to regain your composure. Once you have re-established some balance and perspective, you can come back and face the problem. A brief trip or a change of scene—whenever it is possible and practical—can give you that new perspective. There are times when everyone needs to "escape"—even if it is just a respite from routine.

The answer is
peace of mind

The end result of balanced living should be peace of mind, though it will be made up of different ingredients in different people. Peace of mind is within reach, but it requires thought and action. It is the one sure and abiding answer to the evil of stress and tension.

In the specialization that is required of most people today, many have forgotten in part how to live. Many are no longer well-rounded people with a broad appreciation of life. Joy in sunlight, birds, and flowers is left chiefly to the poets; delight in line and curve is left to the artist; drama and make-believe belong to the stage. But enjoyment of all of these is the right and privilege of every one of you and is a vital contribution to both your mental and physical vigor.

The fit man can depend upon his body and mind to remain fresh throughout crowded days of work, through patience-trying conflicts, through all critical periods. But this fitness can only be maintained by mental alertness that detects stress and offsets it, that recognizes tension for a debilitating state and releases it, that sees worry as a fruitless expenditure of energy and conserves power by taking wise action about all problems.

Everyone of you has a ration of one body with one set of organs to last you for life. This body, if it is to serve out its span without unnecessary wear and breakdown, must be treated with simple mechanical understanding. It is not a feeble, perishable weakling. It can be pushed far—very far—and it can most often find resources to recover. But why place strain upon it needlessly?

The impacts of adversity cannot always be avoided, but if you permit the stress of these impacts to continue without taking rational steps to relieve it, you suffer uncalled-for damage.

Index